Praise for
Defining The New Normal

Colleen is a teacher we can all learn from. Her book can guide you on your journey through the troubled times you were never prepared for. It is truly a guidebook created by an exceptional coach and contains strategies easy to apply to your lives, as she has done. You will both learn and benefit from her experience and guidance, easing your challenges on your journey through life.
~Bernie Siegel, MD, Author of *The Art of Healing and Faith, Hope & Healing*

I love every single bit of your book. The questions you ask are just so incredibly insightful, relevant, and helpful to achieving a better understanding of where we are in the illness process, and how we can improve that. It gives us patients some power and control. Are we going to choose a healthy life in support of our best health and well-being? Are we going to be pro-active in our own care and be our own best advocate? Which steps do we need to take to make that happen?
~Cathleen Frelhofer (Patient)

If life is pure potential, "Finding the New Normal" is pure motivation. Colleen's book is a hands-on, step-by-step manual for taking control of your mind, body, and spirit. Read it, work with it, and take the life-changing action steps you need to re-shape your own destiny and thrive.
~Timothy O'Connor (Editor)

This book is great. The questions helped shed light on areas in my life that need attention. I can tell this is going to be a kind of workbook, which will continue to help every time it is read. The fact that a lot of your questions can be applied to life in general (with or without illness) makes it even better!
~Diane Ramirez (Patient)

"*Defining the New Normal* is informative and enlightening, and is written in a style that is easy to read. This book is based on the author's life experiences as a certified holistic health coach and educator, as well as a patient of a chronic illness. Anyone with a critical or chronic illness looking for answers and hope, or is attempting to support a loved one going through health issues, will find this book very useful."
~Lyle Ernst (Author/Editor)

I really liked the book! It was very thorough and succinct. My favorite part was the defining moments at the end of each chapter. I believe those will engage the reader and help him/her evolve. They will also have fun doing them as they are easy (but meaningful) and to the point. I actually cried when you spoke of your defining moment that led up to implementing the plan with the pharmaceutical companies. It was a great example of empowering oneself and helping a lot of other people.
~Tiffany Gunderman (Patient)

Defining
The New Normal

A Guide to Becoming
More Than
Your Diagnosis

Colleen Brunetti, M.Ed., C.H.C.

Bannon River Books

Please Inquire About
Multiple copies for support groups
Other bulk purchases (25+)
Guest appearances and keynotes
Guest blogging and articles

Address inquiries to the author
Colleen Brunetti
coach@colleenbrunetti.com
(860) 833-9788
www.DefiningTheNewNormal.com
www.ColleenBrunetti.com

ISBN: 978-0-9908842-0-0
eISBN: 978-0-9908842-1-7
Library of Congress Number: 2014953873

October 2014

Jacket Design and Photography by:
Greta Lindquist-Merlino
Linden Tree Artistry
http://www.lindentreeartistry.com/

Printed in the United States of America

ABOUT THE AUTHOR

Colleen Brunetti started her career as a teacher, but after the diagnosis of a critical lung disease (Pulmonary Hypertension) in 2008, she was forced to leave the field. Faced with possible death, and almost certain disability, Colleen began a journey to re-invent herself. Implementing a holistic lifestyle, which included both conventional medicine and alternative care, she began to heal. She eventually far surpassed every medical expectation, and in ways that could not be attributed to medication alone.

Colleen became a certified health coach and now teaches other to do the same – to thrive, not just survive with critical disease. Colleen has traveled the country speaking to doctors, researchers, and patients, and has spoken formally to the FDA twice on her experiences. In addition, she has pioneered a project that is revolutionizing the specialty pharmacy industry for her disease.

Colleen's other interests in health coaching center around supporting busy moms and educators. She teaches stress reduction and lifestyle modification techniques that allow clients to reach their wellness goals, from weight loss and better eating, to more life balance and tranquility. Colleen loves to support those who make it their life's work supporting others, especially parents and educators.

Colleen resides in Connecticut with her husband and young son, a cat, a dog, and together they await a pending adoption placement for a little girl.

You can follow Colleen's health coaching work at
www.ColleenBrunetti.com

A very special acknowledgement of gratitude to the Caring Voice Coalition, who took a chance on an unknown writer, and offered their generous support to make this book possible.

Thank you so much for believing in this project.

www.CaringVoice.org

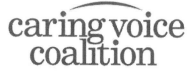

Dedications and Thanks

To the patients who inspire me everyday.

To the Pulmonary Hypertension Association, who gave me the first tools to "thrive, not just survive", and then pushed me to my limits (and then past them), in what I thought I could do to pay it forward and also make a difference.

To the family and friends who hold me up, hear me out, and make me laugh.

To my "Writing Party Buddy". Oh yes, we totally rocked this. I can't wait to read yours.

To my middle school English Teacher – my Dad. Who first told me when I was twelve years old and wasn't ready to pay attention that I should be a writer, and then brought things full circle by also serving as editor of this book.

To the one who taught me compassion and the gift of listening – my Mom.

To my brother and sister. Because you're you and we're us and that's the best.

To my husband who held down the fort through many late nights and long weekends of writing, and who always stays my home base as I rush about.

To my reasons for living – my children, present and future.

I love you.

TABLE OF CONTENTS

TO BEGIN
Introduction
How to Use This Book and What to Expect

TO BEGIN

Introduction

Welcome. I am so pleased you are taking the time to read this book. Perhaps you are someone newly diagnosed with a chronic or critical illness, looking for answers and hope. Or perhaps you have lived with one for some time and need a bit of a re-boot. Or maybe you are looking at this book in an attempt to better support a loved one going through health issues that sometimes can be very difficult to understand. Whatever your reason, I am glad you are here.

Since 2008, I have lived with an illness that comes with a host of descriptors: chronic, critical, debilitating, progressive, incurable... you name it. The picture being painted is (was) very bleak. Does that sound familiar?

The thing is, I have learned that all these labels really mean exactly... nothing. They may seek to describe a disease, but they do not describe you. They cannot describe the journey you will go on. They cannot describe your outcome. Let me repeat that. *They cannot describe your outcome.*

The reason for this is simple. You have more control over the outcome of *your* life, even with this illness hanging in the balance, than you can ever realize. Ever.

Why "ever"? Quite simply, because life is constantly shifting. New things come up, and old things fade away. Some of these shifts will be good, some not so good, and a few will probably be earth shaking. Still, even with so many outside factors, you remain in control. True, you may have to re-calibrate from time to time, find new ways to stay in control, but such is the journey.

The outcome of whatever you're facing actually depends on what you do with the control you have. Do you take it? Do you grasp on to it with a passion and determination that defies logic and expectation? Or do you relinquish it and cling to that ultimately meaningless list of medical words, statistics calculated on people who are not you, and the outcome of others?

I suggest you do the first. Resolve right now, before reading any further, that your journey through this book is the point in time where you take control of your own destiny with the illness you have. If you already feel you have already taken steps to do that, then bravo. You're already on your way to ensuring you are more than your diagnosis. That you have a disease, but it doesn't have you. Now, prepare to take on some more. There is always more.

I do not claim for a second to have it all figured out. I will learn something new tomorrow. I will end up flat on my face time and time again. My illness will likely throw me a curve ball that leaves me reeling... for a time. But I hope that the stories I tell you here, the steps I ask you to take, and the changes I challenge you to rise to and meet, result in just one thing. You, in the driver's seat, the author of your own tomorrow, no matter what your medical chart currently reads.

Are you ready? Let's get started.

How to Use This Book and What to Expect

This book is based on my life experiences as a "professional patient" and also as a certified holistic health coach and educator. In it, I strive to bring you concrete professional guidance for a path to wellness (which you will create!), along with real-world stories, illustrations, and applications.

The book is arranged to take you through a series of lessons and activities that will help you accomplish several crucial steps to understanding how to "define your new normal" as a patient, and to develop a series of self-care skills that ensure you are the one choosing your path as a patient.

In almost every chapter you will find a "Defining Moment". This is your opportunity to begin to explore how you might put the concepts introduced into play in a way that works for you. Feel free to write in this book and mark it up to your heart's content. Alternately, I've created a booklet of "Defining Moments" in PDF form and they are available to you on the website: **www.DefiningTheNewNormal.com/book-downloads.** Use the code word **NewNormal** to access the page, a little gift for you, the readers. Once you have the booklet, print it out and use it over and over, as much as you'd like. By printing the booklet, you'll always be able to re-visit the activities and apply them as needed, for the moment you are living in, long after you've put this book down.

As far as book organization, and the journey we will take together, we first start with getting clear on your diagnosis story which is directly related to how you now define yourself as a patient, and how that sense of self allows you to move forward, or perhaps has been holding you back. You will really need to have a solid understanding of how you feel *now* as a patient before you can begin to work on areas targeted in this book, and ultimately move towards greater strength and overall wellness. We all start somewhere, and it's important to be kind to ourselves in understanding where that starting point is, how we can learn from it, and then begin to move forward.

We then move into your life as an empowered patient. The goal is for you to take control of your medical experience, from how you interact with your doctor, hospital, insurance companies, specialty pharmacies and any other involved parties, to the choices you make in your care and medication protocols.

From there, we move into my favorite part: you as YOU. Aside from the doctor's appointments, and the time spent on your medical care in other ways, who are you? How do you make sure that while you have a disease, it doesn't have you? We'll take a good look at all those things that make up who you are, mind body and spirit, and how you can learn to nurture yourself in radical ways so that you are as strong and healthy as possible *while* you navigate your diagnosis.

All of these things work together in a symbiotic relationship. Each has a place. Each will have a time in life in which they might need more attention than the others, and that's fine. The goal is simply to move forward, focused on taking care of yourself, and you'll be doing it right.

Consider this book a primer of sorts. Each chapter will give you good information to get you started in thinking about your care and sense of self, and you may be introduced to some new concepts along the way. They're meant to be starting points for you, to get your feet wet (so to speak) in many different ways in which you can really care for yourself. If you love an idea I hope you choose to go deeper into it using local resources near you. Or get in touch with me and we'll see about some distance coaching. Let this book be your jumping off point, and you choose how far to go and where to land.

You will be asked at times to perhaps step out of your comfort zone, and to try some new strategies. I invite you to welcome the challenge! There's nothing too crazy in here, I promise, so just give some of the ideas a try. If after giving it your best, you find an idea that is truly not for you, that's okay too. Just think about the big topic you're being asked to consider and find your own way to put it into action.

And that's it, really! Go through this experience with an open mind, and with the ultimate goal of learning to care for yourself in a way that helps you feel better and be a little stronger inside and out. You are a fighter, and so worth investing in, and I thank you for letting me be with you on this piece of your journey.

PART ONE

Defining The Journey

Chapter 1
Not Just a Day - The Months When Time Stood Still

Do the difficult things while they are easy and do the great things while they are small. A journey of a thousand miles must begin with a single step.
~Lao Tzu

My introduction to the world of chronic illness seems to have begun sometime in 2007. I was 28 years old and had been married to my college sweetheart for six years. We had our son, Aidan, on September 3, 2006. He was beautiful and perfect, and other than a 37-hour labor bringing him into the world, having him had been more or less uneventful.

A teacher by profession, I returned to work on a part-time basis when Aidan was four months old. The next six months or so were pretty typical of a young couple starting out. We bought a house in June of 2007, I started a new school year in my job as a special education teacher that September, and then the proverbial you-know-what hit the fan.

I worked in the lower level of the school, essentially the basement. I began to notice I had trouble navigating the two small sets of stairs to get to the main level. Truth be told, I had some weight to loose. My son didn't sleep well. We had bought a house and moved. So I was over weight, out of shape, tired, and stressed... like so many new moms. Right? I paid the annoying symptom little mind.

But as the fall progressed, I got worse. A little light began to dawn, a nagging voice began to whisper... something is not right.

I had always been quite active. Going to the gym was actually fun for me. I had the kind of stamina and activity level most people would do well to strive for. So, really, it was easy to beat myself up and tell myself that I had a post-baby body and all I needed to do to feel better was to get active.

And then, things started to really spiral. First, it became difficult just to go out for a walk with my son in the stroller; then it became nearly impossible. That fall and winter things continued to decline. I contracted pleurisy three times in a row - an infection in the lining of the lungs that made it so painful to draw a breath I sometimes felt as though I was dying. Naturopathic remedies, antibiotics, repeated trips to doctors; nothing was stopping this thing. Finally, one night I ended up in the ER, having nearly fainted while climbing my basement stairs.

A work-up in the ER yielded little, although they did give me a chest x-ray for pneumonia. It was on this chest x-ray that it was found my heart was grossly enlarged, and I was sent, STAT, to a cardiologist.

Two weeks later, on January 2, 2008, came the diagnosis of Pulmonary Arterial Hypertension (PH). It is a rare, incurable, degenerative lung disease that was also destroying my heart. A disease that, by the current literature at that time, said I had 2.8 years to live untreated, and a 50/50 chance of surviving five years if I took the treatment options, which were expensive and dramatic at best.

My son was 15 months old. I took the treatment options.

Chapter 2
"Welcome to Your New Normal"
(Nothing About This is Normal)

I have so much chaos in my life, it's become normal. You become used to it. You have to just relax, calm down, take a deep breath and try to see how you can make things work rather than complain about how they're wrong
~Tom Welling

What were those days and those months that followed diagnosis like? Some of it is hazy. It was a total shock. To go from being a young mom of a baby boy, quickly climbing the ladder in my career, to lying in a hospital bed staring at words scrolled across a medical chart that were about to change my life was... earth shaking. I had two very distinct reactions, and they happened at the exact same time.

I remember putting on a very brave face for most people around me. I calmly told them what had transpired. I was sick. And it was serious. I would calmly explain what the next steeps would be. I would answer their questions on how I was doing with, "I'm okay." (Absolute crap - how can one be okay after news like that?)

While friends and family were kind, and they did ask how I was doing, I wasn't really ready to articulate anything other than just the facts. Sometimes holding those feelings tightly inside falsely feels safer, even as they erode away your sense of balance and control in the most insidious ways. Just once I told a friend over the phone, *"Well... I'm okay. But trying to grapple with your own mortality is tough."* I heard her suck in her breath and then stay silent for a moment. What could she possibly say? That's the closest I got to being honest with anyone for a long time.

I kept my days pretty normal, focusing on work, family, and friends. But the nights... the nights were a different story. I stopped sleeping well, getting maybe 3 – 4 hours of sleep per night. Lying there in bed, feeling my heartbeat pound in my chest (you are NOT supposed to feel your own heartbeat all the time, thank you!) only served to heighten my anxiety. I would get up, and pace the house, and cry and cry and cry. I was very depressed, and highly anxious.

Eventually, those late night meltdowns began to lessen. The anxiety and depression had a strong hold, but life sort of continued on, albeit with a pretty dark cloud hanging over it. I got lucky too though. I found a group of patients, who had what I had, who understood what I was going through, who helped me through.

One thing patients often say to a newly diagnosed patient is, *"Welcome to your new normal."* A "new normal". What exactly does that mean? Well, when it was said to me, the context implied to me, *"This is how life will be now. Best to accept and adjust. Let us help you. Let some things go. We have ways of coping - and we'll show you how too."*

In short, it was a statement of support. A statement of acceptance. And for that intent, I was truly grateful.

Except I took total exception to the whole thing! Normal? I was 28 years old and staring down death. My baby might not grow up with his Mama. I might not see him get to Kindergarten. I was taking more medication than I could possibly wrap my mind around. I let doctors go in through a major artery in my groin and thread a camera into my freaking heart while I lay awake and watched the whole thing on a screen above my head for goodness sake! And on and on and on.

Normal? No. Not in the slightest. And I certainly was not welcoming it. Can you tell I have some Irish in me? I was as angry about the whole thing as I was scared and in a state of grief. Do you know the feeling?

But, you know what; that mix of anger and fear, that feeling of wanting to crawl right out of your own skin and go find a life that doesn't just hurt so darn much... that's kind of a good thing. Because it was when I got to that stage that I took the first baby steps on forging a new path. I sure couldn't keep living like that. And I was going to have to do something about it.

Now that time has gone on, and I've come to grips with all this and learned how to care for myself so that I can feel better, I know I've learned a lot. In retrospect, getting some professional help at that stage would have been immensely helpful. Now I am determined that whenever I start to feel poorly again, be it physically or emotionally, that I get help sooner rather than later. I'm determined to care for myself mind, body, and soul. I'm determined to reach out to other patients so they don't go through what I did. And I'm determined to teach others that a diagnosis is not end-game, that it is only the beginning of learning to move forward.

My path to wellness will always be an ongoing process, one that loops and detours as life carries on. Yours will too. But like the diamond that emerges from great pressure, the result can in fact be something of a beautiful one. The key is not only learning what works for you, but being in tune with your own needs enough to know when it is time to make an adjustment.

Learning to cope and move forward as a patient really begins with an understanding of where you are right now. Much like the stages of grief, I believe the stages of accepting a diagnosis and creating a path forward takes time and changes as you adjust both physically and emotionally. So, let's start at the beginning, your beginning. Your diagnosis story.

Where are you in your journey? Where ever it is, snatch it. Own it. Feel it. And then use it to propel you forward

Defining Moment

Take some time to get clear on your connection to your diagnosis story. Once you've spent some time working with where you *were*, you are better equipped to work on where you want to get. Journal the answers to these questions.

1) What led up to my diagnosis?

2) How did I feel when I got a name for my disease? *(Was it a shock? Or maybe it was a welcome relief, finally someone could tell you a name for the symptoms that had been plaguing you. Something else?)*

3) What were my emotions around that time? *(They were probably quite complex and involved many layers. They may have even shifted hour-by-hour, minute-by-minute. Write down the range you experienced.)*

(continued on next page)

4) How did I express those emotions? Was I honest with myself? Was I honest with others?

5) What was the initial reaction from friends and family? How did I feel about their reactions then? Now?

6) How did I educate myself about my illness at first? Online research? Seeking out other patients? What roll did my doctor play in educating me?

7) How does my diagnosis story affect me now?

CHAPTER 3
No Expiration Date on My Foot:
Choosing to Live No Matter the Diagnosis
A Four-Step Process

Acceptance doesn't mean resignation; it means understanding that something is what it is and that there's got to be a way through it.
~Michael J. Fox

I got a whole lot of good advice in those early months, a lot of it the same advice I now use to try and comfort others in their early stages of an extreme diagnosis. A sense of humor sure doesn't hurt either. One thing I remember other patients telling me quite frequently was, *"There is no expiration date stamped on your foot!"* Don't you just love that? It's true, of course. We all go out, and unlike that mystery food in the back of your fridge (more on that later, too!), nobody has given us an approximate date to leave this world for the next.

Or maybe it isn't the idea of your untimely demise that troubles you. Perhaps it is the fear of treatments that threaten to drag on forever. The fear of slowly declining. Of losing your dignity along the way. Of seeing no end in sight. Yeah, I've faced all those down too. Still do. They don't go away sometimes. It's part of the package, I'm afraid.

The key is asking yourself, what are you going to do about these fears? Hyper-focusing on what might come to be... well, that really doesn't serve any other purpose than to give you wrinkles. And those come in time, too soon as it is, right? So, let's start to get a handle on those fears and see what we can do to take back control. Here's where to start:

1. Identify It: What is "it"? You tell me. What is it in your life, about your illness, that is keeping you up at night with worry? What is it you try to talk about that causes the anxiety to bubble up, the tears to threaten to spill over? Simply put, what's bugging you? Name it. Put it in a few words, or a few sentences. And say it out-loud. To the mirror, to a trusted friend or loved one. Just name it.

Once you name it, you're going to be able to start to own it. And once you own it, this incredible thing begins to happen... it stops being able to own you.

2. Acknowledge It: Being diagnosed with a chronic or critical illness is some scary stuff. It brings all sorts of crap to the surface. And I promise you this, if you keep pushing things down, and keep pushing them away, they are just going to keep coming back. Even if you successfully stop letting the thoughts dwell in your head, they are going to show up, and they're going to show up in your health: stomachaches, headaches, sore muscles... where do you store your stress? That's where you're going to start seeing these bad boys.

So, as we work our way through this process, understand this: I am not asking you to deny what you're feeling. In fact, I want you to acknowledge those feelings. It is the next step in owning them.

3. Feel It: It's okay to cry. To scream. Call a friend over, pour a glass of wine, and let it all out. Throw something if you must, just nothing too valuable, you know. Give yourself the time you need to really feel what you're going through. You are going through something huge and despite what your friend, neighbor, and co-worker's uncle once removed happens to think and share (uninvited), no amount of deep breathing, yoga, prayer, happy thoughts, or good drugs can actually lessen the *truth* of that. Nope, doesn't work that way. Although make no mistake, these things can truly help you cope along the way, and we'll work on them in a bit. For now though, you need to know that it's okay to feel what you need to feel.

But there's a trick to this.

Do. Not. Wallow. Do not stay there too long.

Acknowledge and put words to those feelings. But then prepare to take steps to move on. Realize you may need to go through this process periodically. Realize you might need some professional help from time to time, or maybe for a long time. There is no shame in seeking help. This up and down cycle is a totally normal part of the journey. Again, it's what you do when faced with these feelings that really counts.

4. Do Something About It: Doing something about where you're at is probably the hardest step. Whether you're reeling from a new diagnosis, or have been feeling poorly for so long, it can be hard to change our thoughts and actions to start a new path.

Diagnosed with Parkinson's Disease in 1991, Michael J. Fox is a leader in the chronic and critical disease community, and one of my personal heroes. The man just doesn't let anything hold him back or hold him down. I don't pretend to know what his hard times look like. I'm sure he has them. But the way he continues to move forward despite the obstacles inspires me greatly.

His advice on how to move forward hinges on the choices you make. In his book *A Funny Thing Happened on the Way to the Future*[i], he says,

"Don't spend a lot of time imagining the worst-case scenario. It rarely goes down as you imagine it will, and if by some fluke it does, you will have lived it twice. When things do go bad, don't run, don't hide. It will take time, but you'll find that even the gravest problems are finite, and your choices are infinite"

Sometimes it doesn't seem we have infinite choices, right? We have the diagnosis we have, the medications available, the cards life has dealt. However, I think infinite choices come into play not only with our actions, but with our thoughts as well.

This is what I call our "inner monologue". Some people actually refer to it as "the inner dialogue", but I don't find that quite as accurate. We have that voice in our head talking to us, giving us messages about what we experience, but generally we don't talk back.

So the inner monologue are those things we are always telling ourselves as we move through life. What we choose to focus our thoughts on, how we plan our day, how we interact with those around us… these things are all somewhat dependent on the stories we tell ourselves in our innermost thoughts. Sometimes those thoughts are at the surface and we are aware of them as we go. At other times, they rest below the surface, but impact our general mood and outlook nonetheless. While the inner monologue can be hard to change (you've been talking to yourself for a very long time!), start here and see how it moves you forward:

"I am having trouble accepting _____ about my diagnosis. If I stay in this headspace and don't do something about it there is a cost. I will continue to feel _____, and that will affect _____ in a negative way. But if I can get my head wrapped around the issue and start working on thinking about my diagnosis differently (or taking steps to feel better), then the benefit will be _____. And that is totally worth it."

What you do at this stage in the process is highly individualized because it completely hinges on what is impacting you, where you find comfort, and most importantly, the effort you put in to move forward. As think about moving forward in this process, know that staying put in a space of discomfort or emotional pain does not serve you. Finding a place of peace or acceptance does. While your choices are indeed infinite, it helps to have a few ideas to get you started.

To establish what you're going to do about the things that bother you about your diagnosis it is also helpful to break this step down into three more sub-steps.

Find Your Why: What makes this life worth living, the fight worth fighting? Whether you have a serious diagnosis or not, we all have those things in our world that make it worth being here. The trick for patients like you and me is to identify those things and hold on tight. Find your "why" for being here, and for moving forward. It might be your child(ren), your spouse or partner, extended family, a beloved pet, supporting other patients like you, or something as simple as the smell of the rain or the sight of the sunset that brings you joy.

Find Your What: What is it you already do, or can do to feel invested and productive in life? What is it you can work for, or work towards to achieve? Do you love to write? To craft? To cook? Do you want to deepen your learning on a topic or learn something new all together. What can you engage in every day? What goals can you set for yourself that give you a sense of purpose?

Find Your How: Okay, you know why you want to make changes. You know what that first change might be. How are you going to get there? Think outside the box if you must. It might take some re-framing of your thoughts. It might take some time to save up some money. It might mean taking a really brave step and establishing boundaries in a relationship or walking away from a personal dynamic or situation that is no longer serving you. These "how" steps are not necessarily easy. But they are worth it.

Fellow patient Regan Sobaje-Pierce found her WHY, WHAT, and HOW in this,

"I have decided I'm still worth investing in. No matter how much time I have left, I shouldn't live it waiting to die, holding off in making any plans to see when I'll get worse. I feel up to working now, so even though I've been a stay at home mommy for five years now, I've started studying for the CBEST test to start my path to becoming a teacher! I'm excited and nervous, and honestly it feels good to have decided to continue to plan and live my life. To not let my heart issues hold me back. Maybe it's part of that whole "new normal" thing they talk about. Hopefully I'm finally adjusting mentally to moving on and not just wallowing in PH."

You can go through this four step process for each challenge you are facing. In addition, you may find you get to a really great place for a while, but then something happens and you need to repeat the steps of acceptance and action all over again. This is totally normal and absolutely okay! In fact, if you get to a place of total peace and never get knocked out, you'd be in some sort of nirvana and you need to send us all an invitation. Otherwise, rest assured you are living the ups and downs of the human experience, and repeat the steps as necessary.

Defining Moment

It is time to take the steps needed to work through some of the feelings around your diagnosis and current state as a patient, and then to really grab on to how you will find the focus that helps you move forward.

1) **Identify it:** What is my big worry or stressor around my disease? (*Yes, you have to pick just one for now. The temptation may be to tackle too many things all at once ~ CHOOSE ONE! Find your path to success in beginning to take control of the stressor, and follow through. You can always come back and repeat this page again for another focus later.*)

2) **Acknowledge it:** Understanding that there is something about this worry that is impacting my health or stopping me from moving forward, I will take time to be present with how it is making me feel. *(Write down how it is impacting you.)*

(continued on next page)

3) **Feel it:** Feel what you need to feel around this worry for a few minutes. What thoughts and emotions is it bringing to the surface? Write them down here. Spend some time breathing deeply as you let the thoughts enter your mind. Don't stay here too long though. Give yourself a set time to spend time in this space (maybe 10 minutes or so at most for this activity), and then take a very deep breath and continue on with the next step. If you want to jot down what this part of the process was like, you can do so here.

(continued on next page)

4) **Do something about it:** Now that you've taken some time acknowledging and understanding this worry, it is time to start addressing it so that you can begin to heal and move forward.

    A. Identify your **WHY** for moving forward:

    B. Identify your **WHAT** that you will work towards:

    C. To establish your **HOW**, write down three action items you can do right now to start to address the worry or to feel better.

        i.

        ii.

        iii.

CHAPTER 4
Re-defining "Wellness"
When "If you have your health you have everything!" loses all meaning

Health is a state of complete physical, mental and social well-being,
and not merely the absence of disease or infirmity.
~World Health Organization, 1948

Isn't it funny how we have these platitudes that get us through? Those sayings that put complex emotions and life-shaking events into a neat and clean little box so that we may properly admire or discard them. "This too shall pass!" (Sometimes it doesn't.). "Tomorrow is a new day!" (And it might still stink.). And of course the biggie for those of us with chronic and critical illness - "If you have your health, you have everything!" (Screw that!).

Once you're hit with a life altering diagnosis, these nice little messages can fade away rather quickly. And that's right about the time we need to turn them on their ear.

Let's take "health". I am a certified health coach. That means my job is to help people find their personal best in wellness. Ironic, right? Especially given that my medical chart has me pegged as in a category of some of the sickest people known to the system (i.e., those with degenerative, incurable, and generally regarded as fatal illnesses). Ah! But here is where we take what we're given and do something about it.

Against all odds, I'd actually call myself a pretty healthy person. To look at my medical chart or to know what my disease is and does, you would probably say, "not so". My heart still looks a little crappy, my disease lives on, my medication price list makes insurance CFOs swoon. But... I am well. See, first I was supposed to be dead. And that didn't happen. Then I was supposed to get progressively disabled. And that hasn't happened. Then the meds were supposed to stop working at some point. Except they haven't.

And all of my doctors now say they expect me to live a long and happy life.

What has happened is simply this. In the past couple of years I went from being critically ill to probably the strongest I have ever been. Why?

This is the funny part - everyone I know can tell me why. And the reasons fall into a few distinct categories.

The medical folks: "*Your medications are working! Yay for modern science!*"

The religious folks: "*God has heard our prayers! Yay for miracles!*"

The alternative folks: "*Medication could never do this! Yay for alternative approaches!*" (And then fill in an insistence on using your favorite cure-all: fish oil, kale, meditations, etc.)

And I sit here listening to all these opinions (one philosophy rarely acknowledging the roll of the next), smiling and nodding, and I just keep thinking... *what if, just what if, the approach to wellness is not a single road? What if the definition of wellness, and the definition of health (meaning the absence of sick) are two different things? Can you be well even if you are sick?*

In a word, yes.

Here's why. On this journey, I have learned so many things. I have learned to allow the value of Western medicine to have a place. But I have also learned to take control (if not downright snatch it sometimes) by being my own advocate. I have learned to listen to my body in ways I never did before. I know what to eat to feel vibrant. And, perhaps most importantly, I have realized my human limitations and acknowledged that there is a spiritual force at work on which I must sometimes lean on and rely, because absolutely nothing else will pull me through.

This is not an overnight process. You just have to start...one step at a time. That is, you have to start if you haven't done so already – if you are a patient savvy enough to pick up a book that helps you blaze your own path, then you are probably already invested in making some changes. You've already taken the first step!

So whether you're really new to this whole self-care thing, or you've been working on it for a while, just focus on however many areas of your life that you can. Is it just one? Fine. Three? Fine. Every chapter right now? Go you! I would need a nap. Keep in mind that what's compiled here took me several years to get a hold on – and I'm still working hard on many areas. So you just resolve to start the momentum and keep it chugging along. I'll guide you through the rest.

CHAPTER 5
Getting Out of the Box

The mind and body are not separate units, but one integrated system. How we act and what we think, eat, and feel are all related to our health. Physicians should be capable of teaching this behavior to patients.
~ Bernie Siegel

Here in America, we have what is considered "Western Medicine", sometimes called "allopathic" or "conventional" medicine. Western medicine is just that; medicinal practice that originated largely in the Western hemisphere. It relies heavily on the scientific method, doctors, nurses, machines, and pharmaceuticals. Lots and lots and lots of pharmaceuticals.

The concept of Western medicine tends to be quite singular in focus, thus we have a specialist for everything. Upset stomach? See a GI Specialist. Chronic headaches? See a Neurologist, and so on.

Many of these specialists are fantastic. The human body is a miraculous, complicated, and dizzyingly intricate system. It is crazy to think one doctor could become a deep expert in the whole thing. So these specialists narrow in on what they know, do their thing, and for that we can be grateful.

But, this system has some serious limitations. First of all, there is the issue of the pharmaceuticals. Don't get me wrong, I'm not anti-meds and I would never suggest you should be either. But go grab that pill bottle you've been prescribed for your condition and check out the side effects. Did you cringe? And let's not forget that for many patients the reality is that they then have to take more medications to combat the side effects of the first medication. It quickly becomes a vicious cycle that can be hard to break.

Here's what I notice. Many of my friends take a medication targeted for specific cells in their lungs and end up with upset stomachs. Or they take a medication meant to dilate the blood vessels in the lungs and end up with chronically stuffed sinuses.

At the very simple level this says one thing. The body is intricately connected. When you target one area, you start a cascade effect that impacts many other (often unintended) areas. The body functions as a whole system. Period.

So, when someone gets ill and goes on a highly targeted regime to attack the illness, two inherent risks emerge. First, there is the unintended systemic-wide consequence of treating the illness. Obviously, these consequences (or side effects) are worth it to, let's say… be able to breath. Or walk. Or get up in the morning. Secondly, with such intense focus on the area of concern, care for the rest of the body kind of gets left behind and forgotten. That part is never worth it.

Although a singular reliance on pharmaceuticals is not my favorite thing, and I wish as a culture we weren't popping so many pills, let's go with the premise that these medications are necessary for function and survival. Goodness knows I see them as such, and if you're reading this book after a major diagnosis, you may too.

But what we don't want to do is just stop at medications and Western medicine alone. Here's how I see it – as was mentioned, when I was diagnosed, the average survival rate for my disease was 50/50 at five years. I was told medications might slow the progression of the disease, and perhaps some of the heart damage I had incurred could be reversed, although, most likely, only temporarily. While the miracle was that there were even medications to begin with (prior to 1995 there were not for my condition), the crummy part was that the best Western medicine had to offer was to buy me a little time - at a big price.

Well… I clearly wanted the time. And I was even willing to pay some of the price. But what I eventually realized was that I could not stop there. Western medicine was a box, and if I wanted more for my life, I couldn't just stop with what was being offered. I had to, as the saying goes, "think outside the box" too.

CHAPTER 6
Embracing the Concept of Holistic Care in a New Paradigm

"In essence, if we want to direct our lives, we must take control of our consistent actions. It's not what we do once in a while that shapes our lives, but what we do consistently."
~Anthony Robbins

It's no secret to my friends and family, and probably comes as little surprise to you as well, that I was, and still am, a fan of alternative medicine. Prior to diagnosis, I didn't even take so much as an aspirin on most occasions. I was great at self-treating for the little things, and quite happily seeing a naturopath for everything else. I didn't even have a primary care doctor who practiced Western medicine. It was "natural" everything, no question.

That kind of lifestyle can go a very long way. But clearly it can have limits too. I don't know about you, but I was raised on tofu and sprouts and homemade yogurt, and I still got PH. All the healthy lifestyle practices in the world were not going to give me a pass on this thing. And it was pretty clear that if I chose to treat this disease using *only* alternative practices, my outcome was looking pretty dire.

I often think that people who insist that the body can *always* heal itself or that all Western medicine is bad are able to say so because they have the luxury of never having lived the threat of having their lives cut short by something incurable. Good for them. I, and so many other people thrown a life threatening diagnosis, are not given the gift of time to try out the smoothies and the supplements and the meditations and the colonics as their first line of defense. And no matter how much I would have rather taken that "alternative" path alone, the truth is, sometimes life is going to throw you the kinds of curveballs that defy your comfort system and force you into new ways of thinking and living.

Therefore, it was imperative that I made this paradigm shift. I had to go ahead and embrace what Western medicine had to offer, and while I did that, stay true to my roots and belief system. I discovered something amazing along the way. Practiced in conjunction with one another, these two seemingly at odd practices can work in a pretty beautiful harmony. The trick is finding the balance between the two, and carrying them both out with consistency.

CHAPTER 7
Wellness From the Inside Out

The part can never be well unless the whole is well.
~Plato

Before we dive into how to integrate a holistic lifestyle into your traditional medical care, let's get a few things straight. First, this book and what you should do with it is about progress, not perfection. In fact, please make that a mantra going forward: "Progress, not perfection." Repeat that phrase often.

Of course, I hope the ideas you are going to explore help you take the power to re-shape your world for the better. But as I said at the beginning, not all the ideas will be right for you, and that's fine. You may choose to work on one, two, or any combination of these things. Some you may need to tackle later. Some you may not be in a place to tackle (yet). That's fine too.

What you do not want to do is to fall into a pattern of stagnation with your self-care. Don't let whatever challenges you're facing make your choice for you – the choice being between moving forward by making efforts to improve, or staying still in a place of discomfort and accepting that as status quo. I find the status quo is rarely as it seems anyway, especially after a little creative thinking.

It's okay to make some changes and then give yourself time to make the changes stick before moving forward (just don't wait so long that you forget you're moving on!). It's okay if you do well, slip up, and have to re-calibrate sometimes.

Constantly remind yourself that you are in control. You always have choices to make. Every decision should be made with the intention of feeling better. If you always keep in mind what is safe for your individual condition, then you're doing the right thing. Amazingly simple at the end of the day, isn't it?

So, let's consider what this journey can look like. I'll continue to share with you my path and you can use what works from it for you to start your own. I know I have always been immensely grateful to learn from those patients who have come before me and showed me the way, so I'll share some of their stories too. As you know, you can consider the suggestions we'll go over, or if necessary, choose a different version for yourself all together. What is going to count is that you move forward. In some way, and every day.

To be clear, this path was not always evident to me. Right after my diagnosis, I have already shared how I was in a downward spiral of depression, anxiety, and grief. I wasn't thinking about taking care of myself in anyway past praying (begging) for survival and trying to wrap my mind around a new medication regime.

But then after a while, a funny thing happened. I didn't die. And I was responding well to medications. And I started really paying attention to the fact that there were plenty of other people doing really well too.

So, there came a point of choice. I could continue to live like I was dying (which is no way to live at all), or I could choose to really live. And if I was choosing to really live, I had to start making some changes about what I put in my body, within my life, and how I controlled my thought process. That's where it really started for me, this path of finding wellness while being by medical definition, "sick".

To begin with, I realized my belief system of what made one "well" originally entailed four things:

- **Food:** What we eat matters. A lot.

- **Exercise:** It counts – no matter how little or how much you can do. And you can probably do more than you think is possible.

- **Spirituality:** Is key. No matter what form it takes for you, be it organized religion, or finding stillness and peace in nature, or anything in-between.

- **Sleep:** Can make or break your ability to cope. And it can elude you like crazy, particularly when stressed or in pain.

After attending The Institute for Integrative Nutrition ® in 2013 to earn my certification as a health coach, my view broadened even further to include many other concepts of what makes a person whole and healthy. Concepts such as finding joy and creativity, getting a handle on career and finances, exercise, my personal relationships, and so on. Together, these kinds of topics make up the concept of "Primary Food"[ii]. From the Institute of Integrative Nutrition® website,

Sometimes we are fed not by food but by the energy in our lives. Modern nutrition – carbs, proteins, fruits, and vegetables – is really just one source of nourishment, which Integrative Nutrition considers "secondary food". Secondary foods nourish our bodies, but are not able to give us the joy, meaning, or fulfillment that primary food provides. We hunger for play, fun, touch, romance, intimacy, love, achievement, success, art, music, self-expression, leadership, excitement, adventure, and spirituality. All these elements are essential forms of nourishment, and the extent to which we are able to incorporate them determines how enjoyable and worthwhile our lives feel.

Put more succinctly, what feeds your soul? What makes you human, and what makes you uniquely you? Along with a good path of self-care in diet and exercise, to learn to be well (no matter the diagnosis!), you have to spend time thinking of *all* of these things, and spend time nurturing them. If you've got a diagnosis that has impacted the way you live, sometimes you have to go outside the box even further and find *new* ways of doing these things.

I started on making changes, working to figure out how theses things were defined under an umbrella of also living with a diagnosis. It appeared there were so many other areas to work on to be *me*, still the same person, but with a new piece in play – my diagnosis. The longer I worked under this paradigm, the better I started to feel. The longer I was diagnosed, the more I realized this would always be an ongoing process too, and that was kind of cool.

To begin on this more holistic path to wellness, it is important that you begin to learn to listen to your body. This is a rather nebulous direction, isn't it? We're used to feeling things like hunger and thirst, but our go-go-go world has made it harder to tune into the more subtle messages we receive. Add in chronic illness factors such as pain and fatigue, and it can feel even more challenging.

When faced with a chronic or critical illness, there's a lot to do in order to start to feel better. You don't have to be overwhelmed by it all though. I can't repeat this enough: Step-by-step, one thing at a time, you can make really significant and life altering changes. What that looks like for you will be highly individualized, and it will also likely need to change over time, depending on the course of your disease. Medication changes, changes in your functioning or health status, life circumstances outside your actual illness (that somehow effect your health anyway)… all of these things can create the need to re-adjust.

In order to do all of this, it takes a lot of self-care and know-how. The required efforts are well worth it, and the skills you can easily learn. In addition, as you have already explored with your diagnosis story, to know how to move forward, you have to be very in tune with where you are and where you want to go. But instead of relying on a broad guideline such as "listen to your body", let's start the process of breaking down things and organizing a plan.

PART TWO

Defining You – The Patient

CHAPTER 8
Your Doctor – Your Team

A doctor, like anyone else who has to deal with human beings, each of them unique, cannot be a scientist; he is either, like the surgeon, a craftsman, or, like the physician and the psychologist, an artist. This means that in order to be a good doctor a man must also have a good character, that is to say, whatever weaknesses and foibles he may have, he must love his fellow human beings in the concrete and desire their good before his own.
~ W.H. Auden

Take a minute to re-read the title of this chapter. *YOUR* doctor… *YOUR* team. Notice what stands out there?

I'm sure you guessed it – there's only one person who takes the lead in the medical team, and that's you. Does this mean that you know better than your doctor, or any other member of your medical team? No, of course not. Those medical folks spent countless hours studying and working to be in the medical field, and they should get their due respect as an integral member of the team you work with.

But you still come first. You're still central to the process. You still get veto power on decisions. However, if you're the leader, that also means that, at the end of the day, you're the one who should be taking the most responsibility. You have the responsibility as a patient to be well informed, to ask questions, to be honest about how you're feeling. You need to be forthcoming about if you're following prescribed protocol, and you have the right to challenge assumptions that don't fit you. You also have the responsibility to rely on the informed knowledge of others.

There are folks in the "natural living" world that eschew doctor advice, or brush doctors off as pill-pushers or cogs in a medical machine. Don't get me wrong, there's plenty of disarray in the American health care industry (that's a whole different book), and there are plenty of doctors who won't be right for you. But there are really wonderful caring ones out there too. And if you're dealing with a chronic or critical illness, you need to find one. In fact, think of it as finding a long-term relationship. You need to find THE ONE.

Things to Look For in a Good Doctor

Even if you've been diagnosed for quite some time, read this section anyway. You might find it's time for a shake-up.

There's a tendency to see our doctors as demi-gods. The be-all-end-all-that's-what-the-doctor-said-so-that's-what-I-do figurehead. It's time we as a society change that paradigm. I believe this is already happening. Patient care is becoming more individually focused, and medicine has the potential to someday be something that can be tweaked to an individual's DNA! On the other hand, we're also facing a time of increased regulation with more demands and paperwork being put on our medical professionals. If we want to keep a patient voice in the medical system, we have to speak up for ourselves consistently.

What kind of doctor is the "right" doctor or the "good" doctor? That depends on a few things. The first is the diagnosis with which you are dealing. Or, perhaps more accurately for many of you, the multiple diagnoses! That may mean multiple good doctors need to be found.

You want the best of the best that you can get. You and your care are worth it. However, you need to be mindful of not only specialty areas in general, but also of target areas of expertise. In other words, a cardiologist can treat a heart, but not any cardiologist can treat *my* heart because my particular heart issue is caused by lung problems. A pulmonologist can treat the lungs, but not just any pulmonologist can treat *my* lungs because my lung problems screwed up my heart. So... I will take someone in either of these specialties, *but only one who is a pulmonary hypertension specialist.*

How about you? Think about the intricacies of your own medical condition. What kind of specialist is right for you?

In addition to doctors themselves, you also need to consider *their* team in the office. You can probably get by if the secretary is cranky or the medical assistant who checks your pulse and goes over your meds is a little dull. Sure, we want these people to be great too (and certainly we need them to be accurate!), but you're probably not going to be spending a whole lot of time with them comparatively speaking. The one person besides the doctor you are likely to spend a lot of time with, however, is the nurse or nurse practitioner. The same might also be said for physician assistants, depending on the practice you're in, although truth be told my experience with them is a bit more narrow.

I happen to think that nurses are what make the medical world go round. They play such a key roll in patient care management, program administration, and just setting an overall tone for your visit and care. I personally see my nurse practitioner more than I see my doctor. I *really* have to like her (and I do)! Make sure the allied health professionals who are managing your case, the ones you will have consistent contact with outside time spent with a doctor, work well with you and for you.

Bedside manner and attitude towards a patient matters – a lot. A medical professional that listens to you, hears your concerns, and offers feedback is the one you want. Every single one of my practitioners runs extremely late in appointments. And guess what… I love that. I love it because when they get to me, I'm not a name and patient ID number on a checklist in their day, I'm me, their patient. I get eye contact and conversation and care in my appointment and those things take time. And I know that if my doctor or nurse is running late, it is because they are the type of medical professional who offers that to all their patients, and someone else is getting the needed attention while I am waiting. So, I curl up in the waiting room with a good book or a trashy gossip magazine and happily chill out. Because I know when they come for me, I'm going to get the kind of personalized care I value.

There's one other thing you really need to be aware of. Your doctors and nurses are likely the most wonderful of people (if they're not – move on). But as they are highly trained in clinical practice, that's where their focus tends to lie. We can't and shouldn't expect them to be experts in *all* things you. We'll discuss the roll of a palliative care team in all this very shortly, but first, the biggest thing to remember is you are the team leader. As such, your very first and most important coping skill, the one you should develop as soon as possible, and constantly refine, is to be your own best advocate.

The rule is simple: If you feel like crap, get help.

Defining Moment

Think about your key healthcare providers. Are they on your team? Are you working with them in the most effective way possible?

1) The key players on my medical team are:

2) These players are right for my medical team because:

3) Is there anything I need to think about addressing with my team so our relationship is working as well as possible?

4) Are there any members of my team I need to think about having a heart-to-heart with to make big changes, or maybe replacing?

CHAPTER 9
They Could Have Been Goliath

The little things, I can obey. But the big things - how we think, what we value - those you must choose yourself. You can't let anyone - or any society - determine those for you.
~ Morrie Schwartz

If one of the most important skills you are going to have to learn as a long-term patient is that of self-advocacy, you need to know how to use it on all levels, in every aspect of your life. Sometimes, this can take on a much larger meaning than you could ever imagine. Sometimes, you have to take on giants such as hospital bureaucracy, fights for insurance coverage, disability coverage, specialty pharmacies. These are some pretty large systems for one small patient to face down!

My personal battle with my giant started back in October of 2010. At that time, I was in a deep battle with my specialty pharmacy company. My medications are of such a high caliber that it makes it impossible to get them from the drug store on the corner. They must be special ordered and special delivered every month. This company was having serious issues with getting my life-sustaining medication to me as promised; and then there was the pivotal moment I will probably never forget.

At the time, I had to sign for delivery for my medications. When the meds didn't show up one day and I had to wait at home *again* the next day, I missed an event at my son's preschool. I was livid. I was on the phone with a department manager (having long since given up on working with the call center reps) and sputtering out my frustration. I'm usually articulate - I was too upset to be at the moment.

Then the manager said, *"I understand your frustration, I'm a mom too."* And in that moment I knew how much **she didn't get it**, and clarity returned. I replied something to the effect of, *"Yes, but you are pretty well promised you will see your children grow up. I'm not* *promised that because with this disease I don't know if I'll live long enough! This mistake made me miss a moment in his life, and I can't get that back."*

Then I hung up the phone and sobbed. To express that fear aloud was more painful than anything else I had to deal with regarding PH or the pharmacy company. It still is.

And then you know what's really crazy? I started to second-guess myself. Like maybe I should just be grateful I can get the meds at all. Many aren't so lucky. Maybe this wasn't such a big deal. Maybe I just needed to suck it up. And then within the same week, I got my wake-up call. A girl who shared my disease, a girl whose story I had followed from the beginning, died.

I sat at my computer, staring at the news on Facebook in disbelief. It was then that I knew that my sense of absolute injustice and outrage was justified. This was my life they were messing with, and I was already fighting hard enough for it as it was. It was my son's life they were messing with because he was expecting his Mama and she couldn't be there because some yahoo in a delivery center screwed up again. That was so far out of their rights it was unfathomable. In short, the gloves were about to come off if I got messed with again.

Well, we eventually got the delivery issues straightened out, and while I still lived in slight unease as I had completely ceased to trust the company, things seemed okay. I tried to forget the angst that had been caused and simmer down.

Then a new mess surfaced. I started a new medication and had an adverse reaction. The way you track an adverse reaction is simple: get the lot number and report it to the manufacturer, which is exactly what was requested by the drug maker. But as it turned out, the specialty pharmacy's distribution protocol at the time was ineffective in that they did not track such things. In other words, I had no way of reporting my adverse reaction to the manufacturer, and thus there was no way to track a potentially dangerous situation for other patients.

To be fair, tracking lot numbers at the point of pharmacy distribution is not an FDA requirement. But I would argue it should be considered best practice and done anyway - especially when the medication in question has the power to save someone's life or quickly kill them if something goes wrong. And as I knew the pharmacy's competitors *were* tracking lot numbers, I saw it as industry standard that absolutely should have been practiced.

Every time I tried to talk to someone to deal with this issue, I got vastly conflicting information. In short, I felt I was either being lied to (probably not the case), or literally no one had a clue what they were talking about... although I do believe they thought they did and had good intentions, there was clear disconnect between information I was being given, and what was actually happening.

It would take another book to explain what this particular battle entailed. I worked on it for months. In short, I ended up on the phone with everyone as high up in the company as I could stalk. My doctor's office wrote a strongly worded letter of protest. I filed complaints with HR for my husband's company urging them to drop this specialty pharmacy from their insurance plan, contacted the biomedical company that distributes the drug and complained to them that their product was being mishandled, and so on.

Still, I felt I was getting nowhere. The misinformation persisted, and I never did get to report my adverse reaction in an effective way.

And then the next pivotal moment came. There I was sputtering on the phone again - this time with people like corporate pharmacy managers and the head of global patient safety for a drug company. And I was repeatedly told, *"You have my phone number, you call me if you have more issues."* And I finally replied, *"That's all well and good, but what is the next patient with problems going to do? They don't have your number. And I don't want your number. I want your company to do their job."*

And I knew - even if I somehow got my own issues straightened out, odds are it would help anyone else were slim. And the thought that other patients were going through this same mess, and that the companies were getting away with this kind of behavior, was unacceptable to me.

As luck would have it, this was around the time of a PH related conference in Boston in 2011. I was in attendance, along with Pulmonary Hypertension Association (PHA) President, Rino Aldrighetti. I told him what was going on, and that I was having trouble getting a certain key person to return my call. He picked up his cell phone and made the call himself - and he lit that person's voicemail on fire.

Rino then asked me to begin to track the time I was spending on these issues, and to write a letter to the Corporate Committee for PHA and express my concerns. This is a committee made up of representatives from many of the corporations involved with PH care, including drug companies and the specialty pharmacies that distribute their medications. I did so, and what became known as THE LETTER went out. I guess it caused a stir... or so I am told.

We have continued to do hard work on this issue in the years since. I began to gather anecdotes of other patients who were facing issues with their specialty pharmacies and to share those stories both with PHA and with the pharmacies themselves. I feel strongly that the more stories I was able to share, the more our case for reform was strengthened.

Something really kind of amazing happened as a result of all this. These *huge* corporations sat up and took notice. They not only listened to the complaints and concerns, they began to take action. One company flew a team to PHA headquarters twice to meet face to face to address the concern. Major players in the industry stepped up and said they saw our concerns and they were going to have a hand in making things better. These companies are huge. We could be completely beholden to them. However, because there are good people involved, and because our message was organized, polite, to the point, and clear, and because we didn't back down, what could have been a huge fight instead became a team effort.

A Specialty Pharmacy Advisory Board has been launched for PHA. It is comprised of: a patient (me), a caregiver, representatives from specialty pharmacies, representatives from drug companies**, The Pulmonary Hypertension Association**[iii], and **The Caring Voice Coalition**[iv]. We have a dedicated page on the PHA website where patients can self-report issues they are having, and ideally see resolution. This form also allows us to track trends, which can be immensely helpful when the Advisory Board meets. We've identified and discussed in detail the issues at hand, and we're making really positive progress as a team to build on strengths and to address issues.

We'll talk more later on how getting involved can move mountains. This situation is a perfect illustration of how being engaged on many levels can make all the difference. I had already put in a lot of time volunteering for PHA before I took on rolls of formal leadership. Thus, I knew Rino and he knew me. Approaching him and trusting him to help was easy. Had I not seen him in person, I just as easily could have picked up the phone.

I was involved with my patient community. Because of that I cared enough to want to help others besides myself. Because of our relationship, they trusted me enough to carry their stories to people who could offer that help. I used my strengths as a writer to get my message across to the corporations in the beginning, and was strong enough in my advocacy skills to keep after the people that mattered until we started to get somewhere. The end result is that real change has happened.

This isn't some superwoman act. There is absolutely no reason you can't affect the same caliber of change. Remember, getting diagnosed with a chronic or critical illness may have dealt us a really lousy hand. But we are never victims unless we allow ourselves to be. All those years ago, as I sobbed in my driveway after slamming off my phone, I never would have dreamed that such progress could happen. But it has. And it can for you too.

Your giant may not be specialty pharmacy. But I feel that as high-caliber patients, we also are pretty much bound to have some pretty high-caliber challenges we're going to need to face. How you face those challenges down is going to have a huge impact on your outcome. Are you up for it? Here are a few general tips to help you succeed. This list is also available for download on the book website, **www.DefiningTheNewNormal.com**

Top Five Tips for Working With Your Giant

1. Stay in touch: Make sure your contact and billing information is up to date with your specialty pharmacy, doctor's office, hospital, insurance company, and anyone else who might impact how you receive care. Return any reminder calls for ordering medicine, answering billing questions, or making appointments promptly. Follow-up quickly with any questions you might have. Keep a list of all pertinent phone numbers handy.

2. Keep Good Notes: Consider *always* making a note about any conversation with anyone on your medical team (doctors, nurses, pharmacies, etc.). A dedicated notebook that you keep by the phone, in a purse, in the car, or that you bring to appointments can really help you stay organized. This way, if questions or problems do arise, you have a quick way to access what was said and by whom. This consistent note taking is especially helpful in the early diagnosis stage when you are still learning the names of medications, considering treatment options, getting tests, and so on.

Should you run into problems with any company you find you have to deal with, definitely start keeping a log about all contact you are having with them. Include whom you spoke with, the date and time of the call, and any information that was exchanged. If any communication is done via email, print and store the email with your phone notes. This collection may come in very handy during a problem-solving stage when you have to refer to what has happened, or present evidence of what you've experienced.

3. Stay Organized: Keep an up-to-date list of medications, supplies, and dates for re-order. While it is often customary to expect a reminder call for medication re-fills from a specialty pharmacy or for a doctor's appointment, be prepared to take the lead on being ready to make it happen if you are concerned about a low supply of medication or timing of an appointment.

4. Know Your Rights: Have a good working knowledge of your insurance plan, disability coverage, expected co-pays, pharmacy shipping policies, and any other pertinent information you might need. When something changes, be sure you have a detailed (and reasonable) explanation as to why.

5. Don't Accept the Status Quo: Call centers are funny places. You have someone on the line whose whole job it is to interface with customers, many of whom are none too pleased about something! The person taking your call may have a limited scope of information, depending on their training. They may or may not really understand your disease. They probably have something of a script or protocol they must follow. All of this adds up to the simple fact that they might not know about how to best solve your problem.

So, if you get an answer you don't like, or if it doesn't make sense, if it doesn't meet your needs, don't be afraid to speak up and to go higher up the ladder. When I am facing an issue with a company I very politely, but very firmly, refuse to speak with a first-line call center representative at all. Instead, I request a manager the minute someone picks up the phone. I get their name and their extension. Then I put steps 1 – 4 above into play every time. So far I haven't found a problem I couldn't solve by implementing these steps. Not that it's always an easy or quick fix, but it certainly can be done.

Defining Moment

While there may not be immediate action you need to take against your potential giant right now, it doesn't hurt to plan a little bit in case an issue does arise.

1) Who are the "giants", the corporate players, in my medical journey? *(List all the organizations, and companies who impact your wellbeing.)*

2) Are there any current issues I feel like I need to be addressing? What are they?

3) What steps can I take today to start seeing some change?

4) How will I implement the "Top Five Tips for Working With Your Giant" list when working to change things for my best interest?

CHAPTER 10
The Myth and Reality of Palliative Care

*"Nourishing yourself in a way that helps you blossom in the
direction you want to go is attainable, and you are worth the effort."*
~Deborah Day

The concept of palliative care is an emerging one. It didn't really
exist a decade ago. I think the focus on the *whole* patient is a really
exciting one, and one of the best directions modern medicine is
taking right now. But there's a lot of misunderstanding around the
form and function of palliative care as well.

According to WebMD.com[v]: *"Say 'palliative care' and most people
imagine cancer patients being made comfortable in an end-of-life
hospice setting. But palliative care is actually a new medical
specialty that has recently emerged -- and no, it's not the same as
hospice. It doesn't serve only the dying. Instead, it focuses more
broadly on improving life and providing comfort to people of all
ages with serious, chronic, and life-threatening illnesses....Typically,
a palliative care team includes a physician, nurse, and social
worker, Meier says. But it often involves a chaplain, psychologist or
psychiatrist, physical or occupational therapist, dietician, and
others, depending on the patient's needs."*

I love the palliative care model. It really gets at the heart and soul of
what a whole person focused medical management approach can
look like. What I notice is that each of these specialty areas really tie
into many of the topics we are going to look at in this book. To me
this message is loud and clear – there are many parts that must come
together as you seek to be well within a paradigm of also dealing
with a diagnosis. You have to attend to many different parts of the
body, and coordinate efforts too. The needs will vary, from patient
to patient, and even from time to time for an individual.

While by the definition of palliative care a team related to the
medical world provides services, I would also say that you can do a
lot of this team building approach on your own. Since palliative care

is still an emerging field, the responsibility may in fact be yours anyway.

To see where palliative care can fit into your overall wellbeing, try out the exercise in the next *Defining Moment*, then consult with your doctor and do some research on local resources to begin building your own customized comprehensive professional support structure.

As you continue through this book, you'll also get a chance to explore a lot of these areas in much more detail, and work to see how you can apply them in your own life – either on your own, or with a connection to a team of practitioners.

Defining Moment

Take a few minutes to take stock of where you're at with your holistic care that the professionals can provide. Do you need to advocate for help in a particular area?

Use the chart below to help you plan. Fill out the side on the left with the area you would like help in, and the side on the right with up to three resources you can contact to see if they are a good fit for your targeted area of need.

I need help with:	Possible resources are:
	1. 2. 3.
	1. 2. 3.
	1. 2. 3.
	1. 2. 3.

PART THREE

Defining You - The Person

CHAPTER 11
The Case for Good Nutrition

Eat food. Not too much. Mostly Plants.
~Michael Pollan

As we begin to look at all the things that make you "you", let's start with the one thing everyone always wants to talk about, but most find incredibly challenging to tackle - food.

You'll likely notice the topic of food is one of the most lengthy and detailed parts of this book. The reason for this is the targeted idea that you make a choice on how you impact your health every time you eat. That's maybe three to five times per day where you have total control over how you choose to nourish yourself, and more specifically, nourish the body that is fighting a difficult health battle. That's roughly 84 – 140 times *per month* and 1,008 – 1,680 times *per year* that you impact your wellbeing, just by what you pick up with a fork or reach for in the fridge. What an awesome opportunity to do your body good… or damage.

Food Biology 101

The food you eat impacts every function of every cell. It matters. I think this is such an amazing phenomenon. Just think, something as simple as what we eat can be as profound as life changing.

Consider the function of the digestive system itself. Not only does it have the very big job of breaking down our food choices, but it also must then send those extracted nutrients all over the body to do their jobs of keeping our organs functioning, cells reproducing, blood flowing, and energy steady.

Your body is constantly regenerating itself on other very complex levels. Think about if you get a cut. Blood first rushes to the area and clots, forming a scab and protecting the wound. Then skin cells begin to regenerate and grow over the area, creating a new patch of skin (perhaps with a scar). It's pretty miraculous, actually. And what feeds our body the nutrients it needs to build this blood and cells? What we eat, of course!

In addition to these basic biological functions of the gut, there are some lesser-known functions that are absolutely vital to our wellbeing. For instance, our immune systems, which those of us with a serious diagnosis *really* need to be in good shape, are largely housed right in the gut. In fact, according to Dr. Natalia Shulzhenko of the University of Oregon[vi], our intestines contain more immune cells than the entire rest of our body. There is also a delicate play between good bacteria, or microbes, keeping down the bad and keeping us healthy. As Dr. Shulzhenko states, *"There's an increasing disruption of these microbes from modern lifestyle, diet, overuse of antibiotics and other issues."*

We won't be tackling the personal choice between you and your doctor around medications that directly affect your gut bacteria, such as antibiotics, but modern (read: stressful) lifestyle and diet absolutely count as a part of this process too – and those are things you have a lot of control over. What you eat contributes to how healthy your immune system is and how healthy it can keep you. We're kind of making a mess out of our systems, and a lot of it has to do with food.

Trouble with gut health is often linked to food intolerances, which can be sneaky little buggers to figure out. That's because food intolerance doesn't show up like a food allergy[vii]. With a food allergy, you would likely have an immediate and probably fairly dramatic reaction, such as the anaphylactic shock experienced by some people after exposure to peanuts. A food intolerance, on the other hand, is much more stealthy. The effects can build up over time; the sense of feeling poorly may come on gradually, or be almost impossible to link to food. For instance, you might have achy joints or a runny nose, things you would attribute to age, or seasonal allergies, or a cold, and any of these can actually sometimes be linked to what you eat!

In conjunction with food intolerance is the idea of gut permeability or "leaky gut", which is just as great as it sounds. Over time, and with the barrage of poor nutrition and environmental toxins, itty-bitty tiny holes can open up in the lining of the gut, allowing particles to disperse into the blood stream. The body senses these particles as foreign and mounts an immune response, which over time can cause quite a bit of damage. One of the biggest suspected culprits in this cycle is gluten.[viii] There are other leaky gut issues related to other foods and to environment as well, but often gluten takes the lead, particularly when autoimmune issues are present.

I know going gluten free is crazy trendy right now. There are a lot of potential pros and cons, and to know if going gluten free is right for you takes some research and testing. Just know this: If you struggle with any sort of auto-immune condition or unexplained symptoms (such as joint and muscle pain, skin irritation and rash, mood alterations, headache, etc.), consider consulting with a qualified health coach or naturopathic doctor to see if going on a healthy gluten elimination diet or getting food allergy or intolerance testing is a good route for you. Remember that beyond gluten (and also dairy), there are many other foods that are prime suspects and also not-so-common culprits for food intolerances. It is absolutely worth looking into to see if they might be impacting your overall wellbeing.

Emerging research is also looking at the connection to how healthy our gut and digestive system is in relation to our moods and psychological wellbeing. According to Dr. Jane Foster[ix], an associate professor in the Department of Psychiatry and Behavioral Neurosciences at McMaster University and a member of the Brain-Body Institute, St. Joseph's Healthcare in Ontario, Canada:

"Gut microbiota has been linked to behavior, to stress, and to stress-related diseases. Changes in gut microbiota may influence risk of disease, and manipulating microbiota may provide novel ways to intervene in clinical situations related to mood and anxiety disorders."

While science is still working on this whole gut-brain-mood connection, there's some pretty great emerging evidence that the health of our digestive system directly impacts how the rest of us functions. If you are concerned about the health of your gut and the impact from what you consume (food and supplements), you can look into ideas such as probiotics, the use of fermented foods, or such programs as the GAPS[x] protocol, or The Body Ecology Diet[xi] to learn more. Remember, any overhaul of your diet and supplementation, especially to address a known or suspected medical imbalance, should only be done under the care of a qualified practitioner, well versed in gut healing, and with the knowledge and go-ahead from the doctor treating your primary diagnosis as well.

You do not want to risk dietary overhauls that may impact how your body responds to medication without the whole team on board. Even though I am trained in this kind of thing, I still don't start supplements or make major changes without a check-in with my specialist's office. It's just not worth the risk. Of course, I've found myself a doctor who understands the value of holistic care and supports my endeavors, and so it's usually an easy ask and a satisfactory answer, which is exactly the goal.

The Importance of Food Education and Your History

In this section, I am going to encourage you to get support around your nutritional intake, but I am not going to give the usual disclaimer and ask you to talk to your doctor! This is because the nutrition training for the average doctor is at an unfortunately very low rate. They simply do not get the classroom time and experience in medical school to adequately address their patients' nutritional needs. As stated by the American Academy of Family Physicians:

According to the preliminary results of a nutrition education survey conducted in 2008-09 by the Nutrition in Medicine staff at the University of North Carolina at Chapel Hill, or UNC, although most medical schools offer some form of nutrition education, only one-quarter require a dedicated nutrition course.

Moreover, the survey found, the overwhelming majority of schools fail to adhere to a recommendation from the National Academy of Sciences (books.nap.edu) 'that a minimum of 25-30 classroom hours in nutrition be required of all students during the preclinical years,'

followed by reinforcement of that nutrition instruction during
clerkships, electives and postgraduate training.

In fact, the amount of nutrition education that medical students
receive is so 'inadequate' that 'medical school graduates feel
unprepared to intervene in their patients' care with regard to
nutrition,' according to the UNC preliminary survey results.[xii]

Of course, if your doctor has instructed you to watch your sodium or monitor your intake of dark leafy greens because you're on blood thinners, or any other medically mandated dietary restrictions, by all means, do that. I'm not saying don't listen to your doctor's advice, but I am encouraging you to look further for additional resources.

I also hesitate to recommend consultation with just any nutritionist or dietician. Unfortunately, food industry giants such as Coke and Hershey heavily sponsor the certifying body for registered dietitians, The Academy of Nutrition and Dietetics[xiii]. Coke is even going so far as to offer continuing education units to dietitians and doctors on topics such as sugar consumption[xiv].

This presents something of a conflict of interest in the industry. I don't know about you, but I don't want my nutritional advice coming from the soda giants, whose primary purpose in life is to sell sugary and chemical-laden drinks. To be sure, there are plenty of excellent certified nutritionists out there who can help a lot of people – this is not a statement against the profession. Just do your homework on their individual philosophy prior to taking their advice. Or stick with someone with a more holistic bent, such as a health coach. Look for someone whose professional affiliations are not sponsored or at least not influenced by corporations with an agenda.

I think it is completely worth every second it takes to get educated on where our food comes from, what we should consume, and why. The importance of being well versed in your nutritional intake is especially true when you have a big diagnosis to contend with. Most of us don't have a cure in our sights just yet, and because our bodies have to work much harder than average just to maintain energy and functioning, it seems well worth it to feed it as well as we possibly can.

Even though food itself is relatively simple, for many people making healthy choices often is anything but. Food can be incredibly complex to address. For the average person it can be just because old habits die hard, the hyper-driven dieting industry has confused the daylights out of you, or you just don't know what to eat to feel well. When you also have a diagnosis to contend with you may be grappling with additional issues such as fatigue, medically necessary diet restrictions, physical challenges, and a limited income. These are big challenges, to be sure, but they are not all together insurmountable.

Probably the biggest challenge to eating well, when for a long time you have not been doing so, lies in your mindset. My theory is that food is like religion. We adhere to a certain style of eating (much like worship – or no worship) because of a complex set of personal values and circumstances. These can be hard to shift, even if the end result is really good for you. But it is not impossible!

The first thing you want to do is to begin to identify what your value system around food actually is, and how your personal circumstances impact how you live that value system out. You'll get a chance to do that in the *Defining Moment* shortly. First, let's further establish why you're going to want to do this.

Why Food Matters

Although you may make food choices based on certain cultural preferences, generally most of us in America consume what is known as the Western or the Standard American Diet (S.A.D). The acronym is telling – the quality and quantity of our food intake as a nation is sad.

In a S.A.D diet, there is a disproportionate amount of processed foods, carbohydrates stripped of their nutrients, artificial everything (color, preservatives, etc.), and too much consumption of animal products. The average intake of healthy and whole plants-based foods is generally much lower than even government-recommended guidelines. We suffer from a severe case of "portion distortion", with the size of our servings and meals getting larger and larger. In short, the way in which we generally eat is unhealthy, and we as a nation are unhealthy because of it. According to the Center for Disease Control Website:[xv]

Obesity is common, serious and costly

- More than one-third (or 78.6 million) of U.S. adults are obese. *Obesity-related conditions include heart disease, stroke, type 2 diabetes and certain types of cancer, some of the leading causes of preventable death.* (emphasis mine)

- The estimated annual medical cost of obesity in the U.S. was $147 billion in 2008 U.S. dollars; the medical costs for people who are obese were $1,429 higher than those of normal weight.

Re-framing this from the prospective of someone fighting a diagnosis, there are a number of diseases out there that are preventable with good diet and lifestyle, and a lot of these diseases are linked to what we eat, including obesity itself, heart disease, and diabetes. The data from the CDC tells us that those diseases, when you get them, are crazy expensive.

You have a disease that you may not have been able to prevent, and you're paying dearly already, both physically and probably financially. Does it then make sense that you should be as proactive as possible to stay healthy and free from the preventable diseases so that you can focus all your energy and strength fighting the diagnosis you got that it doesn't seem you *could* prevent? I think so.

I cautiously say that some diseases *seem* like they can't be prevented. That's because while we don't have hard and conclusive scientific proof telling us some of today's prevalent diagnoses are preventable or reversible by diet and lifestyle, there is some extremely interesting incoming research that suggests we have more impact and power over our wellbeing than we might have previously realized. Thought leaders in the integrative wellness field, such as Dr. Mark Hyman[xvi] and Dr. Andrew Weil[xvii] certainly think so. Doctors such as this, who practice integrative or functional medicine, make a strong case for not only diet, but also lifestyle practices as the foundation from which we can fight a myriad of illness.

In admittedly complex and rare disease states, the answer to why these diseases manifest isn't so clear. There are great theories on genetic expression, and the concept of epigenetics (where environmental factors may switch gene expression off and on), and of particular interest with this chapter, this idea that food can impact the course of a disease. This is by no means a comprehensive list, but you should know that diseases such as Multiple Sclerosis[xviii], Lupus[xix], and many more, all have really smart people applying modern scientific research to the very old-fashioned idea that you are what you eat. There are many studies now, and many more to come. Some are in mice models (and therefore not yet able to be solidly extrapolated out for humans), some were small studies that would need to be repeated on a larger scale for statistical accuracy, and many indicate the further research will be needed. But I believe we are looking in the right direction.

Can diseases really be cured by food and lifestyle intervention? I would be very hesitant to just use the word "cure" as that's a pretty big promise to make, but I do in my heart of hearts believe people of *all walks* and many disease states have the potential to feel better, and maybe even have some symptoms alleviated simply by what they put in and on their bodies. I think that's a pretty great place to start, don't you?

Defining Moment

Spend some time thinking about the following questions and jotting down your answers. You may be surprised with what you discover about yourself.

1) What was my food intake like as a child? What kinds of food did I eat? When did I eat it (parties, feeling sad, feeling happy, as a reward, etc.)?

2) What kinds of food do I eat now and why? Are my choices impacted by what feels comfortable and familiar? In what ways?

3) Have I made new choices in how I eat recently? Why is that?

(continued on next page)

4) Do I feel like my desire to "eat well" and my ability to do so are at odds? Why is that? Finances? Energy or physical ability to cook? Knowledge of which foods would benefit me most? Something else?

5) What do my hunger signals look like? Am I able to differentiate between true hunger and a feeling (such as boredom or stress) that causes me to seek food?

6) What changes would I like to make to my eating? Can I do it in small steps or is there a really pressing reason to do it all at once? What is my first step towards change? My second?

CHAPTER 12
What's on the Menu?

Life expectancy would grow by leaps and bounds if green vegetables smelled as good as bacon.
~Doug Larson

A key concept to consider when thinking about your diet is the idea of bio-individuality. In simple terms, your biology is unique to you. A dietary concept originating from the Institute of Integrative Nutrition® the idea of bio individuality simply states:

There's no one-size-fits-all diet – each person is a unique individual with highly individualized nutritional requirements. Personal differences in anatomy, metabolism, body composition and cell structure all influence your overall health and the foods that make you feel your best. That's why no single way of eating works for everyone. The food that is perfect for your unique body, age, and lifestyle may make another person gain weight and feel lethargic.[xx]

So, what you won't find from me, as a health coach, is a recommended way of eating that works for all people, and certainly not within all disease states. In other words, I'm not going to tell you that going gluten free, vegan, Paleo, or Space Man is what's best. I'm kidding on that last one, there is no Space Man diet… yet. Give the diet industry time. We're due for "the next big thing" any day now, and space is, after all, the final frontier.

In all seriousness, I would have to know so much more about your individual world to even begin to tackle recommendations on foods that fuel your body best. One of the above-mentioned choices might just be perfect for you, or maybe you need something quite different. What we *can* do right now is look at some overall good general choices that will work well for everyone. And in order to make those choices, you need a little information on what your body uses (or doesn't use) different foods for.

When I first started trying to get well, I changed my diet with one thing in mind: choose a heart-healthy lifestyle that let me control my weight as best I could (even when exercise was not feeling like an option), and do everything I could to make my body as strong as possible while fighting PH. I didn't think I could fix my lungs with a good salad, but I was quite sure I could make life easier on my heart and tummy by following well-researched dietary guidelines. For me, this meant landing on a vegetarian and gluten free diet. I feel so good when I eat this way that it is absolutely worth the fuss of finding and preparing the foods necessary to maintain what is admittedly a bit of a complicated regime.

Besides just feeling better, I'm very confident in the science behind these two eating choices that I'm making personally. This doesn't mean they are the right choices for you because, as discussed, we are each so different. But for me, the research is showing that there are benefits to the way I'm eating even far past how I feel on a daily basis, so I'm investing in my long-term health as well as reaping the short-term daily benefits of having more energy and stamina. It's a win-win.

How are *you* going to choose what to eat and why are you going to be making these choices? When it comes to choosing exactly how you want to eat, there are some other basics everyone would do well to follow. In fact, I am so confident that these are the keys to good nutrition that I want you to copy these down and paste them right on your refrigerator. Or, visit www.DefiningTheNewNormal.com and download the free poster I have for you there.

If you follow these guidelines to the best of your ability each and every time you reach for something to eat you will be doing something great for yourself. You don't need the latest fad. You don't need a television doctor's "amazing- wonderful-breakthrough-secret", you don't need to stare longingly at someone else's before and after photos. You certainly don't need to starve yourself and for the love of everything, skip the "diet" products in every isle. You just need one thing - to understand your body and what it needs to eat to feel well.

The No-Fail Eating Guidelines for Everyone

- Eat more plants
- Resolve to eat better to feel better
- Be open to trying new ways of eating
- Avoid falling into trends – make sure the choices you are making make sense for you, and not what's easy to jump on to based on the latest food fad du jour
- Choose whole foods over ones that are processed
- Be mindful of your food sources – where food comes from and how it is prepared counts almost as much as what you actually choose to eat.

Author Michael Pollan also has this valuable advice,

Once, food was all you could eat, but today there are lots of other edible foodlike substances in the supermarket. These novel products of food science often come in packages festooned with health claims, which brings me to a related rule of thumb: if you're concerned about your health, you should probably avoid food products that make health claims. Why? Because a health claim on a food product is a good indication that it's not really food, and food is what you want to eat.[xxi]

What does this mean, exactly? First let's take a look at this term "foodlike substances" Pollan mentions. Most foods found in a box and often a can or package are so far removed from their original ingredient source they can barely be called food anymore. They're highly processes, artificially "enhanced" (questionably) with supposed nutrients, and are often colors found nowhere in nature, thus more "foodlike", than food at all.

To make these foods seem healthy and worthy of your valuable shopping dollars, the front of the packages are splashed with lovely health claims and pretty pictures. Nutritional buzzwords such as "low fat", "high fiber", "whole grain" and "natural" grace the front. Yet when you turn the package over and really read the ingredients list you may find the supposed good does little to outweigh the concerning, such as sugar content or highly processed and artificial ingredients.

Also beware "green washing". It's super popular right now to make foods (and cleaning products and cars, and so on) seem very eco friendly, even when they're not. The issue is that many of the terms advertisers use are not regulated. The word "natural", for example, has no standard meaning. Crude oil and opium are natural substances too, but you wouldn't eat them! Don't just go by a pretty label, make sure you really understand what you are buying and consuming.

With the words of warning out of the way, let's move on to portion sizes and different food categories, and how to make wise choices within each.

Be mindful of serving sizes: Portion sizes have increased dramatically over the last couple of decades. From actual dinner plate size, to the fact that restaurants now serve food four times the size they did in the 1950's[xxii] you need to be mindful not to fill a whole plate when serving up food. For instance, in-home dinner plates used to be a few inches in diameter smaller than they are now, and our collective waistlines seem to be moving right up with these changes.

A great trick for remembering what an actual serving size is lies in getting yourself a good visual aide. Try picturing common everyday items to remind you what a given portion looks like.

1 TBS – a poker chip (butter, peanut butter)

2 TBS – a golf ball (hummus, dried fruit, cheese, dressing)

2 oz – shot glass (nuts and seeds)

3 oz – deck of cards (meat)

½ cup – tennis ball (ice cream, cooked beans, grains, pasta)

1 cup – baseball (milk, soup, chili, cooked veggies, yogurt, fruit)

2 cups – 2 closed fists (raw veggies)

While it's a good idea to take a little reality check now and then and track your food for a few days, I'm generally not a huge fan of counting calories and measuring out food in ounces and cups. Not only can that make you a little crazy, it also doesn't teach you how to listen to your body's signals or focus on eating more of the good stuff. That's why simple visuals like those referenced above are helpful. And thank goodness there are some basic rules of thumb that help you make good choices at any table.

Instead of thinking of restricting yourself, think of "crowding out". Try eating a little less of the food that isn't in your best interest, and a little bit more of the food that is. Eventually, if you slow down and eat mindfully, you'll have less room for the food that's holding you back from being your healthiest possible.

As far as what to actually eat, consider these following guidelines when making your choices.

NOTE: *While there are people who need to limit or carefully monitor intake of certain foods such as leafy greens if you're on a blood thinner, or certain grains if you're wheat or gluten free, there are general guidelines you can pull from as you make choices within the confines of what is best for you.*

Give plants center stage: Try to fill half your plate with fruits and veggies at every meal. When you do this you not only reap the vast benefits of phytonutrients (the nutrition in plants), you also crowd out some of the bad stuff. It's harder to eat a huge serving of pasta if you've filled up on a good salad first! If fresh is hard to get, use frozen. Avoid the canned varieties of veggies and fruits for the reasons if possible (more on that in a few moments). Remember, fresh is best!

Aim to eat a rainbow every day: In other words, choose fruits and veggies of all available colors. The colors in produce actually reflect some of their varied nutrient health properties, and you want to take advantage of all Mother Nature has to offer in this area. From cancer fighting properties, to a good dose of vitamins, to enough fiber to keep things moving, fruits and veggies keep our bodies as happy and healthy as possible while we fight a diagnosis – eat a lot of them.

Proteins – A bit of a complex choice: Aim to fill about one quarter of your plate with your protein choice.

When it comes to meat and dairy as sources of protein, less is more. Give some careful consideration to how much meat you eat and how much you actually need. According to the Physician's Committee for Responsible Medicine (PCRM), we tend to take in much more protein than our bodies actually need. Further, PCRM states that diet too high in protein can contribute to such issues as: osteoporosis, cancer, impaired kidney function, heart disease, and weight-loss sabotage.[xxiii]

From arsenic in chicken, which has been associated with cardiovascular disease, type 2 diabetes, cognitive deficits, and adverse pregnancy outcomes[xxiv], to the questionable way factory-farm animals are raised, not to mention the abhorrent treatment of animals and the environment, factory farm sourced meat deserves a careful look before you decide to consume it[xxv]. In addition, all meats that are further processed (cold cuts, hot dogs, etc.) are likely to be quite high in sodium and contain ingredients that carry other health concerns.

While from a philosophical point of view I strongly believe that either a little carefully sourced meat, to perhaps no meat at all, is the way to go for most people, there are absolutely those of you who will choose to or feel you need to keep meat as a main player in your diet. I get it! I'm married to an omnivore who l-o-v-e-s his hamburgers. Even he has learned to thoroughly enjoy the more plant-based cooking I do at home though, and he's lost 30 pounds in part because of it, so there's hope for everyone!

When you do consume meat, go for leaner options. Choose chicken breast, lean beef, pork chops, and fish over anything processed, such as cold cuts, or cuts high in fat. When preparing the meat, broil, steam, or bake it. Avoid breaded and fried varieties whenever possible. The negative affect from the empty calories in the breading and the quality and source of the oils[xxvi] in the frying process far outweigh any possible nutritional benefit from the meat.

Give some thought to dairy consumption. There are several things about our love affair with dairy that are, well, a little odd. We are the only species on earth that routinely drinks the milk of another species. We are the only species on earth that consumes dairy past infancy. Milk is meant to fatten up baby cows and make them grow quickly. Past our own childhood growth period, there's no fattening up and quick growth most of us need!

If you're concerned about your calcium intake for strong bones, consider that there are many other great sources of calcium, including (but not limited to): dark leafy greens, broccoli, almonds, tofu, and figs (to name a few!)

Don't get me wrong I know cheese tastes awesome. So does ice cream. There's actually a really fascinating reason we are so attached to our dairy. According to Dr. Natasha Campbell-McBride, author of the book *Gut and Psychology Syndrome*[xxvii], when you consume dairy, the protein casein is absorbed into the body, including the brain. The part of the brain that assimilates these proteins are actually opiate receptors. That's right, dairy makes you feel good because on a biological level you are having an opiate response. This is why Grandma always recommended that glass of warm milk before bed. It really does have a sedative affect. The casein in dairy is meant to lull baby cows down to rest and make them feel good so they want to keep nursing (i.e.: drink milk) As you may have also guessed, opiates in any form are addictive. Those of you who joke that you are "addicted to cheese" really truly may be, especially as the casein in cheese is more concentrated than in some other dairy products. Like any addiction, it can be hard to break free, but it is possible.

While you may still choose to indulge in dairy, give a little extra reflection as to whether you are taking it in because of a perceived need, or a preferred feeling of satiety and familiarity, or an indulgence, and then make your decision accordingly. Nothing wrong with a little indulgence now and then, as long as you really understand what it is you're indulging in.

When considering protein sources, don't discount plants as a great source as well![xxviii] Nuts, seeds, legumes (beans), and even quite a selection of dark leafy greens pack a good protein punch. In fact, one hundred calories of kale or broccoli each have more protein than some 100-calorie equivalent selections of red meat! True story!

Fats - A little of the good stuff goes a long way: There was a time when fat got a really bad rap. If you remember the low-fat craze from the 1990s, where suddenly everything was fat free (and highly processed and packaged!), you know what I mean. This was probably one of the biggest disservices we could have done for ourselves. Foods that are created to be unnaturally low in fat also tend to be higher in sugar, salt, and artificial fillers so that you can't taste how bad they actually are! It's a pretty simple trick of the food industry, actually.

Fat is not in fact bad for you. Our bodies need fat to function. The key is to understand that not all fats are created equal. There *are* bad fats. Generally, these are the saturated fats, which can raise overall cholesterol. At most keep these kinds of fats to 7 - 10% of your diet.[xxix]

Trans fats, fats that have been hydrogenated to withstand food industry preparation and extend shelf life are of particular concern. They both raise "bad", or LDL cholesterol and lower "good, or HDL cholesterol. While the FDA has preliminarily said[xxx] that trans fats are no longer "generally recognized as safe" (GRAS), and that trans fats should be removed from foods, that has yet to happen, nor is there a solid timeline on their removal. So in the meantime, watch for them in baked goods, fries, margarine, some creamers, etc.

Good fats are the ones that either lower total cholesterol, or the "bad cholesterol", LDL. Monounsaturated fats (sometimes called MUFAs) include the fat found in nuts, olive oil, avocado, and coconut oil. Polyunsaturated fats are found from sources such as fatty fish (salmon), flax, and seed oils (sunflower, safflower). These are the fats that will help your brain function, lubricate your joints, help your body extract nutrients from plants, fill you up, and make your food taste good. Most of these in their actual oil form should be cold pressed and not heated, so drizzle on after cooking is done and enjoy these in moderation!

Sugar: Life can be naturally sweet: While I am highly suspicious of the fad diets that try to demonize and eliminate a certain food group, such as we have seen happen with carbs and fat, I suspect the current outcry against sugar is a little bit more on target. Sugar is a non-nutritive substance. In other words, there's nothing in it that your body needs to have in order to function. It does not nourish you from a nutritional standpoint.

Therefore, every time you consume sugar you are consuming empty calories, contributing to weight struggles. There is some emerging research linking sugar to alterations in the brain chemistry associated with diabetes, which impacts the production of a brain chemical crucial to blood sugar regulation and even mood modulation (think depression and anxiety issues), and plays a roll in why you may over-eat.[xxxi] All said, it makes sense that if you're going to have sugar, it's a treat that is best eaten in very small amounts of moderation.

The challenge with sugar for the discerning consumer isn't so much the cakes, ice creams and the candy bars, although those are certainly sources of calories that pack on the pounds and should be eaten in moderation, if at all. However, we all pretty much know that when we eat those we are indulging in a treat and taking in a solidly large dose of sugar.

The real problem is that sugar is sneaky as heck and hides in all sorts of places, especially in foods you might not think of. For illustration sake, a supposedly healthy raspberry yogurt from Yoplait® has 26 grams of sugar. By way of comparison, a Snickers® bar has 27 grams.

To put this further in perspective, the American Heart Association recommends six teaspoons (about 25 grams) of sugar per day for women and nine teaspoons (about 38 grams) for men[xxxii]. One snack of a container of yogurt and you've about reached your quota for the day. It's really easy to do, even with foods you might have considered healthy before taking a closer look.

Sugar hides in much smaller amounts everywhere too. Tomato sauce, ketchup, breads, cereals, salad dressings, and sauces often contain the sweet stuff. And while it may not be much per serving, odds are you are rarely eating just one serving of a given food (most of us don't), and the results are cumulative. In other words, they add up over the days and weeks, resulting in the staggering average American intake of 130 pounds of sugar consumed per year.[xxxiii]

That annual 130 pounds of sugar comes at a potentially even higher price when we battle chronic and critical illness. We can't afford extra inflammation, and extra weight is hard on the body. I know staying away from sugar is hard. So hard! I am a sucker for small-batch gourmet ice cream! But I promise if you eat less, the cravings do diminish over time.

To some, it might seem the simple answer is to reach for the sugar-free and diet products. Goodness knows they are heavily enough marketed as a better alternative. Again, this is buyer beware! If you do the research on artificial sweeteners such as Splenda® (sucralose), Sweet'N Low® (saccharin), or Equal® and NutraSweet® (asparatime), you'll quickly find a great deal of conflicting information from many sources. While the official word is that these chemical compounds used to sweeten food are safe for human consumption, many in the health conscientious world, including plenty of doctors and researchers, aren't so sure.

Frankly, I say avoid the stuff at all costs. If it's made in a chemical lab and not derived from nature, I get suspicious. If you don't know what's in it, your body doesn't either. When it comes to anything in a pastel packet at the coffee bar, I think the jury is still very much out on safety and risk. Yes, these items are currently FDA approved. And, as seen with trans fats discussed above, the FDA also routinely has to switch course when new information on food risks becomes scientifically viable. You're fighting a disease; don't make it harder on your body by consuming mystery ingredients.

Now, this isn't all to say life can't be lived sweet! It can, and it should! In fact, our bodies are programmed to crave sweets. The problem is that the sweets we tend to consume are both addictive and possibly detrimental to our health. But that doesn't mean you need to give up all things sweet! Consider using small amounts of natural sweeteners such as raw local honey, maple syrup, and stevia to add a touch of sweet. Sweet fruits and even sweet vegetables can help satisfy the body's natural sweet tooth, especially if you are mindful to choose these healthier options consistently. You'll be amazed at how your tastes may adjust.

Believing that life is meant to be lived and enjoyed, I even think that an indulgent dessert now and then is totally worth it. But *now and then*, not every night, maybe not even every week. The key is moderation, and on a consistent scale. If you can make a very mindful choice each time you choose to have a treat, and start to read ingredient labels very carefully, you can start to make small steps towards big changes.

Cheers to a glass of wine… maybe: The decision on whether or not to consume alcohol when you have a serious diagnosis is a very personal one. Certain conditions and medications may make it prohibitive, and you absolutely should talk to your doctor about specific recommendations for your alcohol intake recommendations, and follow them.

Be aware that alcohol is made up of empty calories, and some drinks, especially mixed ones, can be surprisingly high in calorie count. In addition, while alcohol may be okay in moderation for many people, like sugar, it does not feed your body anything it needs. If you are working towards a healthy body weight, stop and think before indulging.

That all being said, if your doctor gives the nod, I think a nice therapeutic glass of wine with dinner or a couple of drinks with friends has a place in a balanced healthy lifestyle. Of course, you should never over-indulge to the point of intoxication or dehydration (hang over!). Then again, probably nobody really *should* be doing such a thing either, major diagnosis or not.

CHAPTER 13
Eating Well When You Feel Like Crud

We are indeed much more than what we eat, but what we eat can nevertheless help us be much more than what we are.
~Adelle Davis

Perhaps one of the biggest challenges to feeding yourself well when you don't actually feel well is finding the stamina and motivation to prepare good foods. Your finances may have changed due to a change in your ability to work or the cost of your medications, so it can feel like more of a challenge to afford the healthier options. All of this can combine to create something of a difficult cycle to break. You don't feel well enough to cook, so you reach for "cheap" convenience foods. The convenience foods are generally highly processed, full of sodium and probably chemicals, and low on nutrients.

Then, whether it be right away or over time, convenience foods make it so you don't feel well too, but maybe in a different way than your diagnosis is bothering you. Now you have two issues to contend with! I know it can be challenging, but with some pre-planning and a few good strategies, you can start to eat better to feel better.

Choose convenience wisely: There is nothing wrong with a good short cut! If you're too tired to chop fresh veggies every day, go ahead and buy the pre-chopped ones in the produce isle once in a while. Frozen veggies are the next best thing because they are often picked and then flash-frozen right near the field. Canned foods are not something I recommend too often because they often come with a high dose of sodium and possibly preservatives to contend with. In addition, there is concern about the chemical BPA in the can lining leaching into the food.[xxxiv]

Shop in bulk: Big bulk stores do have their merits. Buying a lot of an item at once cuts down on the number of shopping trips you need to take and often saves some money. When shopping in bulk, think out of the big box store too though! Small health food stores, often with a reputation of being pricey, are often actually a gold mine of savings if you shop their bulk section. Spices that will cost you a few dollars per jar at the grocery store may come in at cents on the dollar. Likewise, you can scoop up a big bag of loose oatmeal, rice, or beans from the bulk bin and save greatly.

Shop online: Price compare with major websites and see if you can find some of your staple items online. Not only may you find them at a lower cost online, you will also save the time and energy at the grocery store. (Visit **www.DefiningTheNewNormal.com** for a list of suggested resources.) Local grocery stores sometimes also offer a delivery service so you can get fresh foods to your door as well.

Cook once, eat twice (or more!): When you do feel well enough to prepare good food, go for it with gusto. Double every recipe and make your freezer your best friend. If you make twice what you need, you actually cut your work just about in half because you won't have all the prep and clean-up to do a second time around. When you double your recipe, put aside half for your meal that day and either save the rest for tomorrow or promptly wrap and freeze the second half. On bad days, you have a ready-made healthy meal to pull from the freezer. Toss in a side of simple fresh veggies and you're good to go.

I use this method *all the time* and it has saved my family from one too many nights of yet another bowl of pasta (the only thing my loving husband will make), or possibly cold cereal for dinner.

Another trick is to cook up a large batch of something and then re-purpose it throughout the week. For instance, a tray of chicken breasts, or the whole bird, is going to make a couple of meals. Likewise, a large pot of rice or a batch of beans can be put to use for more than one meal.

Eating the same thing day in and day out can be tiresome though, right? This is when spices become the variety of life! Take that tray of chicken and a big pot of rice. The first night it's grilled chicken that you add some garlic and rosemary to – eat that with the rice and a salad. The next night you re-heat both with a dash of soy sauce and a bag of frozen mixed veggies and it is a stir-fry. For the third night, re-heat it with cumin, chili powder, and garlic and serve over greens for a taco salad! The trick at each meal is to simply add a new spice combination, a big serving of easy to prepare veggies and a whole grain and you have a balanced and delicious dish that you really only had to prepare once.

Eat in Season: Fresh fruits and veggies are highest in nutrients, last the longest in the fridge, and are at their lowest price point when they are purchased in their natural growing season. If you can also get them grown locally, you get extra bonus points. Buy extra and freeze for use in the colder months when fresh seasonal produce is harder to come by. Everything from berries to kale freezes well. Yes, kale! And spinach too. Freezing leftover greens is one of my favorite tricks. If they are on sale or I've purchased too much for the week I simply wash, let dry, and toss in a big zip lock bag. Pulled out later, they can be added to smoothies, soups, and stir-fries with no prep or extra mess.

Your Freezer, Your Friend: When using your freezer for the "Cook once, eat twice" or "Eat in Season" methods, take a little time to get organized. Investing in one of those food savers that vacuum seals your food for freshness is well worth it. They range from full size full priced models, to little hand held devices at a lower price point. Either will work perfectly fine and the selection really depends on your needs and your budget. Because I often cook a very large pot of stew or baked goods and freeze many portions at once, I use the big one. My sister uses a little hand held device and has a small freezer, and that works beautifully for her.

Sometimes it is helpful to prep your food ahead of vacuum sealing. For instance, I'll make a large batch of muffins one day and freeze them on a cookie sheet first. Then I vacuum seal them. This way they don't end up muffin pancakes from the pressure of the sealer. The same goes for things like freezing fresh fruit and veggies in season – if you spread them out on a cookie sheet and pre-freeze, they'll maintain their shape.

Label everything and store in an organized fashion. Meat goes in one section of the freezer, veggies in another, and so on. If you're super organized, you can also keep a running list of what is actually in the freezer so you know when you're running low on a staple or know exactly what your choices are going to be coming up.

Finally, get creative! You'd be amazed what you can freeze effectively! From peeled and smashed avocados to beans, from individual ingredients to fully prepared meals, there are really only a few things a freezer can't preserve for a while. Take full advantage!

It's okay to get some help. If you are at a particularly challenging place in your health journey, it's okay to let friends pitch in a little. There are wonderful websites where caring people can organize meal deliveries for you. This can be immensely helpful if you are undergoing intensive treatments or really just not feeling well enough. Don't worry about accepting the help – you can always pay it forward later. And there are few things in this world that make people happier than feeding a good friend, sick or not.

In conclusion: Eating well when you don't feel well isn't always an easy feat. But as you can see there is a wide array of tips and tricks you can take advantage of. Use some on one day, some another, rotate through and see what you like to do. I promise you, the efforts will be well worth it, both in the short term for your energy and sanity, and the long term for your overall wellbeing.

Defining Moment

Go back and review each of the food guidelines discussed above. Then review the cooking and shopping strategies. Answer the following questions.

1) What did I learn about food in this section that surprised me the most? How does this inform healthy changes I can make?

2) Choose three healthy changes you can make starting now. Not Monday, not the start of next month. Now. It could be around the types of food you choose, how much you eat, or how you shop for and prepare them. Make these three changes concrete and attainable. Write them down.

- Change 1:

- Change 2:

- Change 3:

(continued on next page)

3) What barriers might I come across when trying to implement these three changes?

4) Here are three strategies I will use when these barriers come up so they don't stay in my way. (Follow through and use them.)

- Strategy 1:

- Strategy 2:

- Strategy 3:

CHAPTER 14
Some Things Are Bigger Than Us

Ultimately spiritual awareness unfolds when you're flexible, when you're spontaneous, when you're detached, when you're easy on yourself and easy on others.
~Depak Chopra

What does spirituality mean to you? Spirituality and religion can mean the same thing to some, but I think they can mean two different things too. There are those who cling tightly to the faith of their youth, or a moment of conversion, and for those people a more traditional religion rings true. Then there are those who claim to be "spiritual, but not religious", preferring to let their faith be guided by something other than an established path. And then there are those who adhere to nothing in particular in the spiritual realm.

Science is seeking to understand how the spiritual dimension of our humanity impacts and influences our journey, particularly when someone becomes ill. A small-scale study examining the experiences of individuals with a life-threatening disease found that the following:

Spirituality greatly affected patients' journeys through a life-threatening illness and provided a sense of meaning despite the illness." And that, *"Participants described how their spirituality provided comfort throughout their journey, strength in facing the life-threatening illness, many blessings despite the hardship of the illness, and trust in a higher power to see them through the journey. All participants described a sense of meaning in their lives throughout their experience.*[xxxv]

While I do have my own deeply ingrained belief system, I'm not here to tell you which way is right. But what I do want you to understand without a doubt is that we *are* spiritual beings. Thus, it is encouraging to see the vast array of studies that are looking at this interplay between spirituality and coping with a critical diagnosis. For instance, a study out of Montana State University, which looked at the role of spirituality in the well-being of individuals living with Multiple Sclerosis (MS) concluded that:

Spirituality may have an important impact on the well being of the chronically ill and others. The impact of spirituality for the chronically ill may be evident in its capacity to supply the coping resources that can be valuable tools in promoting hope and managing depression. The ability to cope with illness is an important factor in improving one's physical and mental health status.[xxxvi]

If we are made up of mind, body, and soul (spirit), and the three are inextricably linked, and your spirituality may have an important impact on your well-being, then to find wellness within a difficult diagnosis, you've got to spend some time working on your soul. When I refer to the soul, I'm referring to that thing that is *you*, your inner voice, your deep emotions, what stirs and calms your heart, that inner space where connection happens on a level that can't really be explained. If you've ever had a spiritual experience, or felt an unexplained sudden sense of peace, you know what I mean. If you haven't had that, let's find it for you.

I can understand how there will be people who feel reluctant to participate in this part of the journey. Certainly there are those who have been burned by religion, or never felt a particular draw to spirituality. But, I assure you, if you rely only on medicine and logic when you're critically sick, something will be missing, or at the very least, you could spend a lot of time in a really uncomfortable place seeking or wishing for a sense of peace that eludes you.

When your doctor says, "This is the best medicine can offer", the brain tends to focus only on clinical outcomes or external factors. When these things alone don't make you feel better or better enough, the heart whispers, "There has to be more, right?"

No matter what your spiritual path may have been up until now, please commit to either sticking to it, renewing it, or finding one.

Here are some ideas to get you started:

- Church – keep going, or go back
- Small group in-home meetings for religious studies and fellowship
- Getting daily verses or inspirational quotes sent to your email or phone
- Spending time in nature. Where's your "happy place" – the one you feel most relaxed and at peace? Mountains? Ocean? Somewhere else?
- Letting music sweep you away
- Breathing quietly while letting your mind relax

How about that last one – just breathing? Not what you think of as spiritual? Try thinking of just breathing as a form of meditation.

I think that if I had to choose the single most powerful source of peace, understanding, and wellness, meditation would be it. Meditation can take on many forms. It can be more formal and spiritual in nature, such as the meditation practiced by many religions, or it can be more general. The beautiful thing about meditation is that you can simply make the practice your own, no matter what your religious path or affiliation. The only rule for optimal experience and benefit is that you do it consistently.

To meditate, find a comfortable seated position. You can sit in a chair with your feet on the floor and your back well supported, or sit cross-legged on the ground or a bed. Wherever you are comfortable.

You have several options on where to place your hands. You can simply rest them in your lap, or rest them on your knees with thumb touching index fingers in the more traditional meditation position. Another option is to bring palms together at the chest, in a prayerful position. As you might be just starting out, this is not meant to teach a *specific* meditation process. Rather it is intended to take you on the first steps to what can be a daily practice.

Close your eyes and just breathe slowly. Inhale through the nose, and out through the mouth. If you are new to meditation, start short.

Even a minute or two of silence within yourself can feel incredibly long if you are not used to taking this time for yourself.
It is likely that thoughts will rush into your mind, and this is totally normal when starting out. Try to clear them by focusing your mind on your breathing. If a thought comes to you, acknowledge it is there and release it, bringing attention back to your breathing.

Another option is to choose a mantra to repeat each time these thoughts rush into your head. A mantra is basically a statement of belief or intention. Here are a few to get you started, or you may wish to come up with one of your own.

"I will make choices today that help me feel my best."

"I am in control of my wellness, my disease does not have me."

"Each day is a chance to do better, and I choose to work towards wellness."

Work up to five minutes of meditation. Then to 10 minutes. Try adding a minute each day or two. You can add more if so inclined. The point here is to spend time just being quiet. When we are quiet, it is then that we can hear best.

Defining Moment

Start with some soul searching! Think about these questions:

1) Where am I now in my spiritual path?

2) What do I do now *each day* that brings me a sense of peace? (If you don't currently do anything, what sort of practices might you like to start?)

3) What is a "higher power" to me? Is it a religious figure? Nature? Something else?

4) Where do I feel most connected to a higher power?

5) What can I do, starting now, to foster or strengthen that connection each day?

CHAPTER 15
Movement that Matters

Movement is a medicine for creating change in a person's physical, emotional, and mental states.
~Carol Welch

This chapter will not tell you how to exercise. A major diagnosis affects people on so many levels and in so many different ways. Your abilities and restrictions will be so vastly different from the next person's, depending on where you are now, and dependent on any physical impacts your health journey has brought for you. ***Personal exercise guidelines absolutely must be worked out with your doctor so you can stay safe while you get stronger.***

That being said, I am convinced individuals of all abilities can do *something* to stay active and to improve stamina. No matter where you are at physically, in order to start feeling better, you have to start somewhere. Let me tell you my story around this.

When I was first diagnosed I was in dire straits. Flashback to 2006: As you know, I gave birth to my son, and no matter how hard I tried, I simply could not recoup my previous activity level.

To give a little more detail on what that looked like, it first became apparent something was not right during what was, for me, normal activity level. I was an avid walker, and since I live in the hills of Connecticut, everything was uphill at some time. There was one point where I was out walking with a pregnant friend and we went up a hill, I pushing my son's stroller, while she's bopping along, and I'm sucking wind, and I had this moment of jealousy and a little disgust with myself. She clearly was outpacing me – and doing it pregnant no less!

The second time was a little more serious. Again, out for a walk, with a different friend. We climbed a large hill and turned down to go back. A few steps later I handed off the stroller, and knelt to the ground, feeling horrible in a way that I was soon to grow to recognize. My heart was pounding out of my chest. I was in a cold sweat, I was so sure I was going to pass out. She looked at me in alarm, exclaiming, *"COLLEEN! You're grey!"* But still, I recovered, stood up and shook it off, and we walked along.

Then my regular days became impacted. I would be teaching my 6th graders math and simply run out of air mid-sentence. And I became a master at accommodations to hide my worsening symptoms, like only climbing stairs when I was alone, or studiously nodding and saying, "hmm-hmmm" instead of speaking in sentences to the person I climbed with. I was quickly learning I could not go up a set of stairs and talk at the same time or I would get incredibly dizzy. Another trick I developed was pausing at the top of the stairs pretending I was going in a different direction than my companion instead of really coaching myself to breathe and hopefully not pass out. Sometimes I would go around a corner and lean against the wall or find a bench and just curl over, trying to catch my breath.

I didn't like how I was feeling, and I was blaming myself, which in retrospect was insane. A few months prior to my life-altering diagnosis, I purchased an elliptical trainer. I was going to stop being out of breath all the time. I was going to lose weight and get in shape. I was not going to be a frumpy mom! Except that every time I got on the thing, my heart would threaten to make an escape from my chest and I would be too busy gasping for air and feeling dizzy to continue.

Then my diagnosis came, and I suddenly understood why what should have been easy physical activity was becoming impossible. I just sort of froze and stopped trying to stay active. I sold the elliptical trainer on Craig's List, *"Barely used – great deal!"* We made a rule in my house, *"Mommies don't run!"* I sat on my rear on the couch, figuring I had every reason to, and there I stayed.

A couple of years went by, and a few tweaks to medication came. It appeared I was going to be around for a while. And I was feeling quite good on the right therapies. I was ready to try to exercise again, but after what I had experienced in those early months just before and after diagnosis, I was pretty scared to try.

However, I decided not to let that stop me. I talked with my doctor and nurse about my hopes, and they gave me a safe target heart rate to stay under and some guidelines. I had to wear a heart rate monitor with everything I did at first. As I grew stronger, with the okay from the specialist's office, I got to challenge and expand the limitations they had given me.

I started with the Wii Fit, figuring I could track my progress and it couldn't be that hard to do. Wrong! The first time I did an activity on that thing I ended up on the couch after two minutes, as the world spun and tilted around me, and my heart started it's old escape routine. But when things settled, I got up and tried again. And again. And again. Then I started water aerobics. I didn't have the strength to tread water, so I had to wear a floatie and hang out with my new friends, the little old ladies at the YMCA. They were awesome. Then I moved to walking outside again, yes, eventually even on the hills. This whole process took months.

And finally, I started Zumba. I had danced nearly my whole life. 13 years of classical ballet lessons and more hours in the clubs in college and my early 20s than I'm going to admit. Losing my ability to dance had long been one of my greatest regrets with my disease. I was so scared to walk into that studio and start a class. The owner of the studio took a chance on a pale slow moving girl who promised not to faint on the premises and she let me join – as long as I kept my doctor's information handy for her should I hit the floor, and not in a cute way. And now I dance several times a week – keeping up with the healthy people. And I've finished three 5k events, including the Warrior Dash twice. (I mostly walk them – running is for being chased by real zombies only).

I know I had some pretty big struggles learning to be active again, and I imagine it's not easy to regain strength while going through any chronic or critical illness. First of all, it's just plain scary to move again. You can't help but ask yourself, am I really out of breath because I'm working hard or because I am being foolish and pushing it? Can I really walk that far? Or is someone going to be peeling me off the floor? What if I hurt myself and tomorrow I feel worse than I do today? But can you walk five steps? Tomorrow, walk six. Can you make it around the block? Tomorrow, go three more houses down. Can you walk a mile? Tomorrow, do 1.2 miles.

Suffice to say, I really truly believe that my ability to regain functioning had a whole lot to do with challenging myself and pushing through the fear, and allowing a little discomfort.

You can do the same. Your results will vary, of course. But I know I got here not only by continuing to exercise in the face of the "impossible", but because I was also busy implementing all the other good lifestyle practices this book discusses.

Remember, the best successes come from a multi-pronged approach, where you care for yourself mind, body, and soul. And go easy on yourself. Effective exercise doesn't have to be hard-core cardio and weights. What counts is getting going and making improvements. I'm quite certain that if you start slowly, move carefully, consult with your doctor, and stick to it, you too will see some results that once upon a time you couldn't even imagine.

Bonnie Johnson, a yoga instructor based in Los Angeles, CA shares some great advice on getting started with an exercise regime[xxxvii]. She says that the most challenging aspect of getting started for many people is just the idea that you must make some modifications, mostly because that can be quite hard on the ego, particularly if you were once active and your diagnosis has changed that.

However, what I learned from my own experience, and from what Bonnie shares, learning to modify, as I did with using a flotation device in a class meant for people 40 years my senior, is a form of loving yourself enough to invest in your wellbeing. As Bonnie says,

To exercise, to move, to breath, is to preserve best we can the God given gift of movement and breath – it's a way of giving ourselves self love, taking care...one feels alive! To have that feeling, that movement, that breath - heals us in more ways than one...You are never alone, every human being has something that challenges them in one way, shape or form. We all just need to allow ourselves to be

our beautiful imperfect selves, and allow ourselves to be kind to
ourselves by being open to assist/help/etc.

While options such as water aerobics, gentle walking, and maybe
even some light weights can be beneficial, some of the Eastern
practices such as yoga, tai chi, and qui gong are particularly helpful
for patients with physical limitations. Each can be practiced very
gently and be modified as you need to – even being done from a
chair! It is best if you can find a good instructor who you can trust to
guide you safely, and with whom you are able to connect.

You are doing something amazing for yourself by investing in your
physical health with whatever exercise is appropriate for you. And
the efforts, even the moments where you're not particularly
comfortable (as long as you're safe), are well worth it.

Defining Moment

This activity will help you identify ways in which you can safely increase your activity level. *Remember that all exercise and major lifestyle changes should be done under the supervision of your doctor!*

1) *If you're currently engaging in regular exercise, write down what you do, including activity, duration, and frequency. If you're not currently engaging in any activity, list your reasons why not.*

What is my exercise routine like now?

2) *Based on where you are at right now, identify a physical goal to work towards in the next month. It does not have to be grandiose. You just have to move forward.*

Right now I can:

In one month, I would like to be able to:

(continued on next page)

3) *What sort of action will you need to take to reach this goal? Choose your activities and schedule them into your day. Write them right on your calendar, put them on your fridge, or set a reminder on your phone. Just get them down somewhere where you will see them consistently and follow through.*

My chosen activity is:

These are the days and the time of day that I will do this activity consistently:

4) *Choose a way in which you will reward yourself for a job well done. What will you do for yourself when you follow through for a month and reach your goal?*

My reward for successfully implementing and following through on my goal is:

(continued on next page)

5) Call your doctor's office and inform them of your goal and how you intend to get there. Use this section to write down any feedback you are given, including their guidelines, preferred limitations you should stick to, and any positive encouragement you got.

6) Record your progress weekly.

Week 1 Progress:

Week 2 Progress:

Week 3 Progress:

Week 4 Progress:

RESULT:

REWARD:

CHAPTER 16
Counting Elusive Sheep

"Also, I could finally sleep. And this was the real gift, because when you cannot sleep, you cannot get yourself out of the ditch--there's not a chance."
~Elizabeth Gilbert, "Eat, Pray, Love"

Ah, sweet slumber. It seems there is nothing our body needs quite so badly, but tends to be quite so dysfunctional with, as our sleep. You are either craving it and can't get it, or you need so much of it, it can be hard to function.

Certainly issues like chronic pain and medication side effects can have a big effect on your sleep, and those are issues you should speak with your doctor about. Beyond the immediate impact of your diagnosis and treatment, there are a number of proactive things you can be doing in order to ensure a better night's rest.[xxxviii] You may even find that when you implement these things that you have less of a need for medically supported sleep over time. Here are my top five recommendations that are easy to implement.

1. Go to bed and wake up at a regular time: We have an internal body clock that helps us naturally fall asleep, stay asleep, and wake up. Going to bed and waking up at the same time each night and mornings helps keep that clock well tuned so your slumber is as restful and effective as possible.

2. Shut off the screens one hour before bed: Specifically, backlit devices such as phones and tablets are a potential issue right at bedtime[xxxix]. This is because the particular light they emit mimics the effects of sunlight in that they can actually significantly interfere with melatonin – the hormone our body emits to help regulate sleep and wake cycles. Shut these screens off at least an hour before bed.

3. Make your room dark: Any sort of artificial light can interrupt sleep patterns[xl]. This includes not only more obvious sources, such as the glow from a streetlight or porch light, but also more sneaky artificial light, such as those that comes from power buttons on TVs, or bright alarm clocks. Block all of these out to the best of your ability.

4. Create a bedtime ritual: Begin to prepare for sleep 30 – 60 minutes before you actually turn in for the night. By repeating the same steps each night, your body begins to anticipate that sleep is near and more naturally starts to wind down. Simple routines like washing your face and brushing your teeth are a good start. However, there are several other activities targeted at winding down, listed below.

5. Experiment with variety of calming sleep-aides: There are many calming activities you can do before bed, including things like taking a warm bath, reading a book, or gently stretching. Here, in more detail, are three of my favorite go-to sources anyone can use.

Guided meditation: There are a number of programs out there that offer a guided meditation to help induce sleep. In guided meditation, the listener gets into a relaxed position (lying down ready for sleep is perfect!), and listens to a pre-recorded segment. Often set to calming background music or sounds from nature, the speaker on the recording offers such things as visualizations, stories, and suggestions for relaxation that bring the listener into a state of deep relaxation.

 The trick to finding the appropriate guided meditation really just lies in your personal preferences. Find one with a soundtrack you like and one that is narrated by someone whose voice you find very soothing. Get into the habit of listening to a guided meditation each night and see how it helps you slip into a deep rest.

Deep breathing: Spending time concentrating on just breathing deeply can be extremely powerful for helping ease the body into a state relaxed enough for sleep. According to resources found on National Public Radio[xli], Dr. Esther Sternberg, a researcher at the National Institute of Mental Health, says that the relaxation response is actually a triggering of the Vegas nerve, essentially our "breaks" that slow and calm us. And Dr. Mladen Golubic, a physician in the

Cleveland Clinic's Center for Integrative Medicine, says that breathing can have a profound impact on our physiology and our health. Settle into a comfortable position and focus on inhaling deep breaths in through your nose, and exhaling through your mouth.

Aromatherapy: There are several essential oils that aide in signaling the body to relax and calm down. Scents such as lavender, vetiver, and ylang ylang[xlii] are all excellent at encouraging a restful state. The great thing about using essential oils is that they are generally so safe and effective, with little to no worry about interactions. From the University of Maryland Medical Center:

Researchers are not entirely clear how aromatherapy may work. Some experts believe our sense of smell may play a role. The "smell" receptors in your nose communicate with parts of your brain (the amygdala and hippocampus) that serve as storehouses for emotions and memories. When you breathe in essential oil molecules, some researchers believe they stimulate these parts of your brain and influence physical, emotional, and mental health. For example, scientists believe lavender stimulates the activity of brain cells in the amygdala similar to the way some sedative medications work.[xliii]

Sleep is so vital to your wellness. It not only impacts your energy during the day, but your emotional stability, your ability to cope, your immune system, and your metabolism. It even the foods you eat, because when you're tired you're less likely to reach for or have the ability to prepare nourishing food. Although challenging at times, it's imperative that you take steps to create healthy sleep habits for your overall health.

Defining Moment

Take stock of your current pre-sleep rituals and sleep patterns. How are they serving you? Is there room for improvement?

1) I sleep about _____ hours per night. I do/do not find this adequate for my rest needs. (choose one). My quality of sleep is:

2) When I wake up I feel:

3) Currently, before bed my routine is:

(continued on next page)

4) To improve my sleep I will try these four things. *(List them, and implement one each week for the next month, keeping track of how it goes. If the first works, keep it, and add in the second habit. If one habit doesn't seem to be helping you after one week of practice, it's okay to ditch it)*

Sleep habit I tried:	Dates I tried it:	How it worked: (or didn't)

CHAPTER 17
Finding Your Creative Beat

The comfort zone is the great enemy to creativity; moving beyond it necessitates intuition, which in turn configures new perspectives and conquers fears.
~Dan Stevens

One of the most important parts of our humanity is the ability to be creative and to express ourselves through such outlets as: poetry, writing, dance, music, and art from all media (painting, drawing, clay, etc.)

Now, before you protest that you are NOT AN ARTIST, hear me out! I believe we can all benefit from the arts. Certainly the benefit can come from engaging in an artistic practice ourselves, and most definitely from enjoying them as an observer. Think of how you feel when a favorite song comes on the radio, or you gaze at a painting from a master. Think of how you feel when you read that perfect poem, or get lost in a good book. The arts evoke emotional response from us in deep and powerful ways, and in ways that can even be healing.

Whether you've previously worked with the arts, or even if you never have before, a great way to get started as a patient is through art therapy. Galen Martin[xliv], an art therapist at Memorial Medical Center in Modesto, CA shared the importance of art therapy for her patients. According to Martin, art therapy is juxtaposition between letting go and taking back control. While engaging in creating art, you can let yourself relax, while opening your heart and mind to the artistic process. The outcome of this is almost the opposite of what one might expect – through this process of letting go, you can actually re-gain some control over what your illness has taken from you.

Here's how it works. When you are contending with a major diagnosis, the illness has a way of sneaking into your every thought and action. Remember that little voice in your head, that inner monologue? That voice that's doing all the worrying and planning for you gets pretty loud. When you take time to mindfully disconnect from that, you gain some control back. Art therapy gives you time to relax, and thus renews your strength so that you can take back control from your illness. Remember, you have a diagnosis, but it does not have to have you.

Ms. Martin recommends that you find an art therapist who is open to letting the patient forge his or her own path with art. An art therapist with a prescribed set of rules for how art should be created, or for what medium (paint, clay, collage, etc.) should be used, will more likely stifle creativity and foster frustration rather than healing. On the other hand, an art therapist who enables the creative process through providing a variety of mediums, and allows the patient to explore at his or her own comfort level will be the guide who helps the patient open new doors to improvement, growth, and peace.

Everyone has their own form of art that helps them relax well. My personal escape is music. I can be totally carried away by a beautiful melody or pitch-perfect powerhouse vocals. I also sing, mostly where nobody can hear me! While I've always enjoyed singing, I took it to a new level after diagnosis. Since it is my lungs that are affected, I reasoned that moving air through them in a controlled manner was like exercise. And if that didn't work, I was having a good time anyway. My voice range has dropped because of my medications and on some bad days I don't have the lung capacity to belt out the notes the way I'd like, but it is always enjoyable. Plus, it just makes me feel strong. To be able to hold a note longer and louder than I could a few years ago feels like an accomplishment.

As it turns out, I learned much later that I was actually on to something as far as the benefits go (score one for "listening to your body"). In fact, some hospitals are even beginning to use therapeutic singing classes as a way to offer support to their patients battling lung diseases[xlv]. The common ground between singing technique and the techniques used by respiratory therapists make for a perfect therapeutic approach.

The benefits of singing also go beyond just the possible physical benefits. According to Time Magazine Online, scientists now theorize the following:

...singing is like an infusion of the perfect tranquilizer, the kind that both soothes your nerves and elevates your spirits. The elation may come from endorphins, a hormone released by singing, which is associated with feelings of pleasure. Or it might be from oxytocin, another hormone released during singing, which has been found to alleviate anxiety and stress. Oxytocin also enhances feelings of trust and bonding, which may explain why still more studies have found that singing lessens feelings of depression and loneliness... The benefits of singing regularly seem to be cumulative. In one study, singers were found to have lower levels of cortisol, indicating lower stress. A very preliminary investigation suggesting that our heart rates may sync up during group singing could also explain why singing together sometimes feels like a guided group meditation. Study after study has found that singing relieves anxiety and contributes to quality of life.[xlvi]

The science is great, fascinating even. But I think what really matters is that the power music has that can be felt first hand. Lynn Ottaway[xlvii], a patient with COPD, Scleroderma, and diabetes, shares that during her most difficult moments, music was her lifeline. For 10 weeks she lay in bed, her family sure that she was going to pass away. The only thing that calmed her was music. First, it was the crooning of Andrea Bocelli and then as she felt better, Gloria Estefan singing in Spanish. She can't quite point to why these two artists spoke to her, but what counted was the peace they brought.

Then there are the more tactile arts. Many patients I know take up crafting or beading. These kinds of activities are great because you can often pretty easily teach yourself and the supplies needed are usually fairly affordable (and many stores have awesome coupons if you keep an eye out!).

Jhenna Pacelli, a patient for five years, shares about her artistic endeavors. What I love about Jhenna's story is how many ways she is able to help and be helped by the arts. She not only uses it to be good to herself, but she supports many causes near and dear to her. She shares:

I paint, draw, and make jewelry! It helps me a lot with coping with this disease because I still feel like I have a purpose! It also helps me forget I'm sick and it helps me relax. I have high anxiety too so its nice to be able to have the abilities to do something like art that can help keep me level headed. I've also helped raise awareness for this disease and others. I made a bracelet for a CF event, I've made bracelets for animal rescues to help them raise money for veterinary bills, and of course I've helped make bracelets for PH events to help get donations for research, and patient support. I've also made bracelets for PH patients that I hope can help them cope a little better being diagnosed with this disease. I hope they can look at the bracelet and smile and know they are not alone fighting this![xlviii]

The beautiful thing about the creative arts is that you don't have to have any sort of experience or real skill to get started. What matters is that you just plain start. There are literally 100 different ways (or more!) to begin[xlix]. Paint to music, allowing the flow of color and line to match your mood and the music itself. Ever see the splattered paintings of Jackson Pollack? His work can sell for a cool $140 million[l] – so don't get caught up in technical perfection! Draw a picture in sand, and then wipe it clean. Create a collage using pictures from a magazine, focusing only on using the images of things that make you happy. Write a short poem or story. Blog. As you begin to express yourself, you will find that stress is released, feelings begin to be worked through, and you tap into the joy of creativity in ways you might not have been able to in the past.

Kathy Van Osdale-Levitt is a folk artist[li] who is also a 21-year survivor of Pulmonary Hypertension. She explains how art has become key to her wellbeing as a person and as a patient.

It seems that art was always there for me when I needed it during the most difficult times of my life. When I was a kid, I was left home alone a lot. I was lonely, bored, and scared. I started to draw. At first it was a way to pass the time, but then I started to do it because I loved it. I studied art in high school and college but did not get into painting until after being diagnosed with PH. I really started to paint out of sheer boredom, like when I was young... but then I started to find I loved painting. It became a passion for me, and more than just a hobby. It is something I look forward to doing and it gives me something else to think about other than being sick. Having a creative outlet is so important for the chronically sick person. It let's you feel like a "normal" person. It allows your mind to wander and be imaginative. Anything that is positive and can take your mind off being sick is a good thing.[lii]

And let's not forget the power of writing. It can be so incredibly cathartic to get your thoughts out on paper (or screen!). Whether you maintain a public blog or a private journal, processing how you feel about your diagnosis, and even just life in general, can go a long way in helping you be well. In fact, researchers have found that,

"By writing about traumatic, stressful or emotional events, participants were significantly more likely to have fewer illnesses and be less affected by trauma. Participants ultimately spent less time in the hospital, enjoyed lower blood pressure and had better liver functionality than their counterparts."[liii]

Haley-Ann Lynn, a blogger at **http://phenomenalhaley.wordpress.com** shares how writing gave her a renewed sense of self and a way to cope. She shares,

As a child, all the way into my early teens, writing was something I was constantly doing. I had no grand story to tell, so I was only left to create them about other people. At the time of my diagnosis, I realized I probably hadn't written anything in a good five years, and I didn't think I ever would. But when I finally came to the realization of what I had survived, and the daily mess I was working through from the minute I felt dizzy in the morning to the insomnia/ death paranoia nights, I finally made the connection that I, myself, was a grand story. Not to sound selfish, but surviving a disease is kind of an accomplishment. Writing gave me back a part of myself, while showing who I was, and who I will continue to grow into daily. Writing isn't just my coping; it's my identification. Without my broken lungs, I probably wouldn't have that.[liv]

No matter what medium you choose, one thing is clear, art can be a window to the soul, and it doesn't matter so much how you go about using it to feel better, so much as it matters that you take those first steps to try.

Defining Moment

Take some time to think about the roll the arts and creativity have had in your life, and the roll they might take as one of your tools for coping or feeling better in your diagnosis.

1) My experience with the arts in the past is:

2) The kind of art that makes me happy as an observer is/are: (Music? Museums? Reading? Something else?)

3) One way I can take advantage of observing or enjoying the arts on a more consistent bases is:

4) Did you ever engage in creative expression and have let it go? What did you used to enjoy? Is there a way to begin experiencing that again?

I used to enjoy:

To start experiencing it again, I could:

(continued on next page)

5) If you're new to creative expression, or wish to try something new, what is the first thing you want to try? What do you need to do to accomplish this?

The art form I would like to try is:

6) Envision this: What are you hoping to feel, or what benefit do you hope to get, by engaging in the creative arts? Look ahead one or two months after you've begun practicing a creative craft regularly. What does it feel like?

CHAPTER 18
When the Days Feel Too Dark

Out of suffering have emerged the strongest souls: the most massive characters are seared with scars.
~ Khalil Gibran

The Center for Non-Violence and Social Justice defines trauma in this way:

The word "trauma" is used to describe experiences or situations that are emotionally painful and distressing, and that overwhelm people's ability to cope, leaving them powerless. Trauma has sometimes been defined in reference to circumstances that are outside the realm of normal human experience.[lv]

To me, this sounds like a diagnosis of a chronic or critical illness could easily be classified as a trauma. In fact, according to Rachel Tuckman[lvi], a licensed clinical social worker with extensive training in mental health and trauma training experience, notes that this is exactly the case. Because a major diagnosis can be quite overwhelming, and people can easily get stuck in a cycle of difficult emotions, as well as overwhelming healthcare decisions and management, the definition of trauma can and does apply to a major medical event.

Anxiety and depression can often come out of trauma. As patients, it is absolutely imperative that our mental health is attended to just as closely as our physical health. After all, the premise here is that we are mind/body/soul beings. We must continue to focus on the whole person on this path to wellness.

While this can be difficult to think about, I actually find it sort of freeing. It gives an explanation as to why when after a diagnosis, or after a long time battling, we can feel just so incredibly emotionally crummy sometimes. Many of us tend to be a bit tough on the outside, society having programmed us to always hold it together, to not show signs of perceived weakness, to put on that brave face. But the truth is, when you've gotten a diagnosis that rocks your world, everything changes. Everything. If your body has changed drastically because of a diagnosis. Is it any wonder then that your mind may do the same, if not at least for a period of time?

Depression, Anxiety, and the Patient: Anxiety and depression can be difficult to navigate. That feeling of dread and uncertainty that tightens your chest, furrows your brow, and hunches your shoulders can be hard to shake. Loosing interest in every day activities and persistent sadness can begin to create a cycle where the longer you stay feeling down and out, the worse you feel overall. This doesn't only affect your emotional well-being, it can actually affect your health as well, including your immune system, cardiologic health, and blood sugar balance[lvii]. This is why it is imperative that you stay on top of how you are feeling and be pro-active about making sure your emotional needs are being tended to, including seeking professional help if needed.

Depression is sneaky because the way it works can actually impair you from seeking help. According to Ms. Tuckman, when you become depressed, it is likely that your sense of self worth can decline drastically. When you doubt your self-worth, you begin to doubt that getting help is necessary, or something you even deserve. You can begin to write off your depression because you don't feel you are worth the attention you will need to get better. The can create a vicious circular pattern. The big lie of depression is when, as you are suffering from it, you begin to believe you are not in fact depressed.

Now of course not everyone who goes through a major diagnosis experiences anxiety and depression. However, both tending to occur in critical illness is real, and it is prevalent. In 2013, The Pulmonary Hypertension Association completed and presented a study entitled, *"The impact of pulmonary arterial hypertension (PAH) on the lives of patients and caregivers"*[lviii]. In this study, they were able to show how PH affects the daily lives of patients. Of particular note were the feelings of loneliness, isolation, and general symptoms of depression that were self-reported in a significant number of respondents.

Likewise other studies focusing on a diagnosis such as Multiple Sclerosis[lix], Rheumatoid Arthritis[lx], and many other diseases, show similar trends, in that patients either self-report symptoms of depression or are formally diagnosed with clinical depression along with their primary disease.

This prevalence of depression and anxiety amongst the critically and chronically ill not only comes as little surprise it is also completely understandable. When your world is rocked upside down, it doesn't always come right side up again very easily. Contributing factors such as pain, anxiety over your health, treatment side effects, and so on can greatly impact your day-to-day sense of wellbeing. This is why it is so incredibly important that patients with a serious diagnosis practice radical self care in all areas of their lives, including their emotional wellbeing.

One thing I've thought about a lot is why, especially at the beginning, did my doctor's office not enquire about my emotional state around the diagnosis? I now know I need to take quite a bit of responsibility for that. I would walk into every appointment with my chin up, notebook in hand, ready to talk about all the options and write down progress and next steps. I treated it like a newspaper interview, not the fight of my life. I'll bet I looked pretty darn pulled together most of the time. What they never knew is that more than once, I would smile, say thanks, walk out of the office, get in the car, and all the cracks would burst. I cried my way home way more times than I care to count The most acute depression and anxiety would always start about a day before an appointment (I barely slept the night before an appointment for years), and if the news was bad, it would follow me for days, or even weeks, after.

Now I know I need to take responsibility for my roll in that part of the appointment, that this process requires I self-advocate, and that I bring things up even if I'm not prompted. I didn't show a lot of vulnerability on the surface, so why would anyone think to ask me? We were, quite properly, focused on my cardio-pulmonary system, not my brain and emotions. As Associate Professor of Psychiatry, Harvard Medical School and Associate Psychiatrist, Department of Psychiatry, Brigham and Women's Hospital, Dr. Quentin Regestein is widely attributed as saying, *"The patient should be made to understand that he or she must take charge of his own life. Don't take your body to the doctor as if he were a repair shop."*

To start with managing your own possible mental health needs, you need a solid understanding of what depression is so that if it arises, you can identify it and begin to take steps to address it.

According to The National Institute of Mental Health[lxi], the signs of depression are:

- Persistent sad, anxious, or "empty" feelings
- Feelings of hopelessness or pessimism
- Feelings of guilt, worthlessness, or helplessness
- Irritability, restlessness
- Loss of interest in activities or hobbies once pleasurable, including sex
- Fatigue and decreased energy
- Difficulty concentrating, remembering details, and making decisions
- Insomnia, early-morning wakefulness, or excessive sleeping
- Overeating, or appetite loss
- Thoughts of suicide, suicide attempts
- Aches or pains, headaches, cramps, or digestive problems that do not ease even with treatment.

Should you notice any of these issues as persistent, please talk to your doctor right away and seek help. While I do not like to turn to psychiatric medication as a first line of defense, and highly encourage your first forms of intervention (along with talking to your doctor) are that you seek to practice the kind of lifestyle changes outlined in this book, and engage in talk therapy as needed, understand that medications are available and for some people, necessary. It's okay.

If you are not able to talk to your doctor, do not get the support there you need, or you find yourself in crisis, the Substance Abuse and Mental Health Services Administration has a webpage where you

can enter your zip code and be directed to local services.
http://findtreatment.samhsa.gov/

Of top importance, also as described by the National Institute of
Mental Health[lxii]:

If you are thinking about harming yourself, or know someone who
is, tell someone who can help immediately.

- Do not leave your friend or relative alone, and do not isolate
  yourself.
- Call your doctor.
- Call 911 or go to a hospital emergency room to get
  immediate help, or ask a friend or family member to help you
  do these things.
- Call the toll-free, 24-hour hotline of the National Suicide
  Prevention Lifeline at 1-800-273-TALK (1-800-273-8255);
  TTY: 1-800-799-4TTY (4889) to talk to a trained counselor.

Anxiety is a state of anticipating what is to come, or an uncertainty
around what may be that leads to a persistent state of unrest. The
thing about anxiety though is that is anticipatory, not necessarily
predictive. In other words, what you worry so deeply about may in
fact never come to pass. Of course, this little fact doesn't make it
easy to simply shake a bout of anxiety, but acknowledging it and
beginning to work with it is a good first step

Diane Ramirez, a long-term survivor of PH talks about anxiety as a
form of projection about the future, using only what you have in the
present. She says, *"When we project, we're trying to complete
tomorrow's job with the tools we have today. And those tools you
have today may not be what you need tomorrow."*[lxiii]

This bit of wisdom came at me through the phone during one of my
own freak-out modes (Yeah, I can write about handling this stuff,
and I do handle this stuff, and it is *always* a process and that will
always have to be totally cool… what with being human and all).
And I found her insight immensely helpful. What was I so worried
about that day? I absolutely can't remember. Probably because it

wasn't so bad in the end. But her words stuck with me long after the anxiety subsided and the world righted again for a bit.

It is rarely a given that our worries about tomorrow become the truths of our today. Of course, we have a whole lot of say on whether this is true or not as well. Not only do we have control over our actions that affect our outcomes, but I believe just the act of thinking about something long enough and hard enough can indeed help (or hinder) it as it comes to pass. Is something bothering you to the point of anxiety? Do something about it!

Maybe this action you take is tangible. You may be able to make changes in your choices, routines, or activities that lessen the impact or change the course of whatever it is that plagues you. Then again, you may not be able to do that at all. There are, of course, things that will happen to and around us that are out of our control.

When that is the case, the beauty in this is that you still *do* have control to some extent – and that lies solely in your thought process and where you allow it to go. Remember the section near the beginning of the book on your inner monologue? Those stories we tell ourselves, and the way we frame our thoughts, count a great deal when struggling with anxiety.

No matter the severity or range of what you are experiencing, understand that not only should there be no shame or stigma attached to depression and anxiety in general, but that as a pro-active patient invested in your own care, you need to take steps to tend to this part of your wellbeing just as much as the illness you are treating. Your overall health depends on it. You need to be invested in your self-care either to avoid depression or anxiety, or handle it pro-actively when it does arise. Remember, it is okay if it comes. But you do have to deal with it so it does not overtake you. You are worth that.

Self-Care: It is always a good idea to develop something of a toolbox you can pull from when you begin to have difficult emotions to contend with. Listening to calming music, calling a friend, and engaging in gentle and individualized appropriate exercise can all help. You may have something else you turn to, and that is wonderful, so hold on to it.

The power of breath is another great tool against anxious moments. We've already talked about breathing in relationship to meditation and spirituality, but this is also a tool you can use to calm the inner storms when they come. Concentrated slow and measured breathing can do a great deal to help you simmer down when the anxiety threatens to boil over.

I like to combine breathing with a physical activity that will release stress. Depending on where you are physically, you may choose anything from a slow careful walk to jumping jacks in the kitchen – whatever works for you. Follow the physical activity with 10 deep calming breaths. For an extra boost of calm, add in some aromatherapy as you breath in a sense of peace. Scents that lend themselves well to inducing calm during anxiety include lavender and citrus oils[lxiv]. Similarly, lavender and citrus oils work well as one tool to support yourself during depression, and the addition of frankincense and bergamot show promise[lxv]. The 1-2-3 combination or releasing nervous energy, breathing in calm, and allowing the power of scent to help balance you is incredibly powerful.

Defining Moment

It is time to build your own toolbox for managing anxiety and depression. Using the resources in this chapter, and your own creativity, create the following list.

1) The first medical or psychiatric professional I will call if I begin to experience signs of depression or unmanageable anxiety is: *(list name and contact information)*

2) Three other professional resources in my area that I can tap into if needed are?

3) These are things that help me become calm, or that give me a sense of peace:

a.

b.

c.

(continued on next page)

4) Five pro-active things I can try out if I am working on managing symptoms of anxiety or depression at home are as follows, (remembering that you've already consulted with a medial professional too!):

a.

b.

c.

d.

e.

CHAPTER 19
Grown-up Life as Planned... Or Not

The only person who is educated is one who has learned to learn and change.
~Carl Rogers

Education, career, and finances are all quite linked. One impacts the other in a circular fashion, and all can be pretty deeply impacted when contending with a diagnosis.

Education: What does education mean to you? From the age of five or six, most of us found ourselves in school for quite a number of years. The idea of education as an important part of who you work to become post-diagnosis can seem a bit of a nebulous connection at first, so let's work through a couple of scenarios I see play out a lot.

1) You didn't complete the education level you would have liked and now your diagnosis and perhaps other circumstances have made it difficult to do so now. Or, perhaps you were on your way to pursuing some higher education, and a diagnosis or worsening symptoms necessitated that you drop out.

2) You completed a level of education you are proud of, but now your diagnosis seems to be dictating you can no longer hold the career you worked so hard for.

3) You've been working hard despite a diagnosis, and now maybe you're feeling like your health may be trumping your ability to work as you wished. You're also wondering how much to tell co-workers and supervisors, and when to do so.

It's a complex set of issues, isn't it? Your sense of worth as a productive member of society, your ability to handle your finances or contribute to the family budget, and your sense of identity in a career you worked hard for all can come into play.

If you've never been able to complete your education to the level you've wanted, or would like to further your higher education level and feel the time is right for either of these, consider trying just one or two courses at a time for now, or perhaps attending school online. Community colleges are a great place to get your feet wet in going back to school. They often have smaller campuses to navigate and the cost per course is lower than a larger university.

Online learning is another fantastic option. With most classes you can log in on your own schedule and participate asynchronously - meaning you can do your work, perhaps at the time of day you're feeling best, and it doesn't much matter when anyone else in the class is also working. Generally, this is done within a certain timeframe, usually weekly due dates or something along those lines, as set by the instructor.

If formal education is not for you, but you still want to further your learning, the chances for free education are just about endless. Many independent business owners run blogs where they share free information within their area of expertise. Some colleges, including those such as Harvard[lxvi], offer open courses, meaning you can take Ivy League generated classes online for absolutely free.

And don't underestimate the power in furthering your education in your disease. Becoming very well versed in how your body works as it fights a diagnosis, how your medication impacts you at all levels, and how you can stay as well as possible are all incredibly empowering ways to educate yourself. In fact, reading this book is a form of self-education!

Careers: Navigating the work world while you are also navigating a diagnosis can get pretty tricky. Many people who find themselves in this situation can indeed continue to work. Others absolutely cannot, be it short term or long term. Sometimes you have to find a modified way to continue to work, such as more time at a desk, or flex hours, but it can often be done.

For me, as a teacher, it was a bit tricky to figure out how to modify my career. While I initially left the field thinking I was taking a temporary leave after a big diagnosis and an absolute crap-response from my supervisors when they found out (story is below!), I realized I really couldn't be keeping up after my very active young students nor could I be exposing myself to their germ pool all the time, and still hope to do well. Despite feeling really good most of the time these days, I also still battle fatigue and my immune system can be pretty whacky because of my illnesses. My husband and I feel it is more important I focus on my health and our son rather than risk everything to return to the classroom.

While on a pragmatic level this seems totally sensible, it also broke my heart. Teaching isn't just what I did, it was who I was. To leave that, especially after working so very hard and spending a ridiculous amount of money on my education, was a rotten feeling.

I had to get creative. I took a job as an online college instructor, and that was a position I held for seven good years. Depending on my course load, I could work 10 - 20 hours per week from my couch. I also started my own business teaching baby sign language and training preschools and daycares to implement signing with their young charges. Just a couple hours a week, and I got my kid fix. I've now moved on to writing and health coaching, and I still love that I can work from home most of the time, and spend just a few hours per week out with clients. It lets me take my time getting moving in the morning, never have to ask for time off for a doctor's appointment (and you know there are a lot of those!), exercise, totally crash on the couch if exhaustion hits at 2:00p.m., and still meet my son from the bus with a smile.

If you *do* still continue to work, you will have some challenging decisions to make around what and when to tell co-workers and supervisors. I learned this the very hard way, twice. When I was first diagnosed I was open and honest about my struggle. On one hand, I sort of had to be. Contractually, I was obligated to disclose something as I took "too many" days off around a holiday, and thus had to provide an explanation as to why. And on the other hand, it was just "me" to be straightforward and forthcoming. But then my principal turned out to be a snake about things. He called the department head and told her I was "medically retiring" (I had made no such claim). As spring approached, and despite the fact that I had never missed another day of work post-diagnosis and that I was performing my job to expectations (and beyond), I went from getting a hand-written card of support from our assistant superintendent to receiving demands on whether or not I intended to return to work in the Fall.

I *had* intended to return to work. And then things got super shady. The administration cut my hours, transferred me to a new school, thus extending my commute, and assigned me a child who had to be chased and physically restrained. They did this with the full knowledge I now had physical limitations. Suddenly, I couldn't do the job anymore, despite the fact that I had seven years as a successful teacher, and my ability to teach children was not impacted. When I protested, I was shown the door.

I suppose I could have sued, or at least fought much harder. But I was in that early diagnosis stage. Scared, exhausted, and overwhelmed, it wasn't a fight I really had in me. So I left. This was ultimately probably a situation where keeping more details to myself would have been very wise. It was definitely a situation where I would have been wise to at least go with unemployment compensation in hand. But I wasn't that wise back then. Learn from my mistakes there if you can.

Obviously, I clammed up after that. At that point, I had begun online teaching and I never shared my diagnosis with supervisors or students. It was so much easier to pull off as nobody ever saw me in person. However, complications arose over time, especially as Facebook became more popular and I found myself hiding online from co-workers I would have otherwise loved to connect with. The more active in my disease I got, the more often my name would appear online. I began to worry.

Those worries materialized when a student of mine Google searched me. He found out about my illness because I was active in online advocacy work, and then wrote me about what he had found, clearly not understanding what it was he was reading. It freaked me out pretty thoroughly. With the good consult of some fellow patients, I quickly realized that by hiding my diagnosis the new challenge I was facing was that I was no longer in control of the messaging around my diagnosis - Google was. And that was a problem.

I switched course. I sat down and wrote a long letter to my supervisors at the college, and to the people with whom I had a freelance writing contract. I explained my situation, and then I held my breath. The response was incredibly supportive. My ability to work with these much better people continued and I thrived in my profession - this time because I was honest and open and people were more than willing to work with me.

What a difference in response, right? Obviously, I can't give you really solid advice on how you should handle talking about your illness within your own workplace, because your outcome can vary as much as my two experiences did. I will tell you this though; think long and hard before you speak. Be judicious about how much information you share, and make sure you really know the person you're talking to (and who they might talk to), as well as your rights as an employee.

Defining Moment

Give some thought to your feelings around your education and career right now, and consider where you'd like to steer these areas going forward.

1) In thinking about my current level of education, I feel:

2) Considering how I might further my education, either professionally or around my diagnosis, I should explore these resources:

3) My thoughts around what information to share about my diagnosis at work are:

Chapter 20
Becoming Financially Savvy

Learn from yesterday, live for today, hope for tomorrow.
~Albert Einstein

Managing your finances in the face of a diagnosis can be pretty tricky. There may be a lot of new bills and variables to manage, from co-pays for multiple doctor's visits and medications, to home health equipment, to a change in income because you can't work they way you once did or had planned to do.

While it is no doubt that these can be big challenges to navigate, some short and long term planning will help a great deal. Ronald N. Lazzaro, MBA, CPA/PFS, CFP[lxvii], a Financial Advisor with extensive experience in this area, suggests that those diagnosed with a critical illness embark on both short and long term planning in order to best prepare for what their needs are in the moment, and may become as time goes on.

When a diagnosis hits, sometimes the financial implications are felt immediately, and sometimes they can take a while to come into play. The over-arching impact, however, is that the everyday does change. Assumptions you have made, parameters in which you did any financial planning, and the tools you have to work with change.

While it is highly suggested that you consult with both a lawyer and a financial planner, there are a few things you can do now to begin getting clear on what you'll need to be thinking about moving forward. Mr. Lazzaro suggests that you start with a few concrete steps to begin your new financial planning as a patient. And this process starts with asking yourself some questions.

- Will there be economic loss for myself or for my dependents?
- Do I need to consider going on disability benefits either now or in the future?

- Is there a chance my change in medical status could result in debt?
- What are the various stages I may go through (being able to work for a time, having to cut back or change jobs, leaving work) and when do I think these might be happening?
- What are my biggest financial concerns?
- What are my wishes for my financial state, both present and future?
- What do I want to see happen for my loved ones?

You can use these questions to begin to get a clear picture on both your current financial state and the variations that may come into play as time progresses. Once you have a good idea of your big picture, it's time to start planning for both the here and now, and for what may come down the road.

Short Term Planning: The first thing you want to do is to start with a budget for today. What are your current costs and needs? Things like food, housing, utilities, taxes, and transportation are fairly non-negotiable. Make those your priority. Then consider more discretionary spending, such as: clothing (you don't always have to buy new!), entertainment, eating out, electronics, etc. Get a very clear picture of what money is coming in and what is going out.

Next ask yourself if there are areas in your budget that you can trim. Now is the time to do any saving you can for the future. If at all possible, begin to build an emergency reserve. If you're still able to work, but anticipate a time when that may change, it can sometimes take 3 – 6 months before some insurance plans kick in, and you'll need a pool to draw reserves from during that time.

Take the time to re-visit any policies you have, such as life insurance, short and long term disability plans, and benefits packages. Sometimes employers offer programs that are group policies where no underwriting is required. What this can mean is that in some cases you can get in on a group plan where your individual circumstances, which may have otherwise disqualified you, may not come into play as much. These plans can be priceless and if you can find one that works seriously consider joining.

Long-Term Planning: Longer term planning will pertain to all your legal documentation that you're going to want to have in place to protect your assets, your financial beneficiaries, and your own end-of-life planning.

If you have minor children to think of, this step is especially crucial to help secure their future. Consider what savings and education funds you hope to have in place for them, and what sort of documentation you'll need to ensure they benefit, and that the money you have designated does not get eaten up by your medical bills! Make sure they also have designated legal guardians in place. Better you make these decisions than the state, or a fight amongst family.

Be sure your durable power of attorney, both for your healthcare and for your finances, is legally documented. Should the time come when you can't make a crucial decision, who do you want to speak on your behalf and carry out your wishes?

If there is a chance that you, the patient, may be a financial beneficiary from someone, the game changes here too. You actually may not want a large chunk of cash coming your way as it can create a Catch-22, where you have too many financial assets to qualify for help, but not enough to cover the cost of ongoing medical care. Consider looking into a special needs trust, or designating a trusted friend or family to become a manager of accounts should this situation arise.

In our case, my sister is that person. We are setting things up so that in the event that my husband should pass, where I would normally be the beneficiary of his life insurance, that my son will become the beneficiary via a trust, and my sister would manage the account for us. This way, should the unthinkable happen, my medical bills will not compromise my son's financial future.

Disability: If you think you're going to need to qualify for disability sooner rather than later, then you should also start working on your application sooner rather than later! Disability can take months, even years, to get approval for, and it isn't unusual to be denied and have to go through an appeals process. It's not a bad idea to look around for a disability lawyer or a patient advocacy group that can help you with this process. Many places provide these services for free, or only take a fee once you are approved. Be aware that you can collect disability and still earn some income under the "Ticket to Work" program. For more information, visit **http://www.ssa.gov/disability**.

Other Help: It can be a bit hard to think about for some, but remember that a lot of good people are out there who want to help those who are struggling financially. Applying for SNAP benefits (previously known as food stamps), shopping thrift stores and food banks, and talking to churches and patient advocacy organizations are all resources you can explore.

Defining Moment

Use this opportunity to get clear on your big picture around your finances, and also to begin the first steps in your short and long-term planning.

1) In light of my diagnosis, my biggest hope for my finances is:

2) My biggest fear is:

3) When thinking about possible beneficiaries (spouse/partner, children, family), I want them to get:

4) The short-term impact of my diagnosis on my financial situation is:

(continued on next page)

5) I envision that the long-term impact of my diagnosis on my financial situation may be:

6) I have the following documentation in place to ensure my financial future, and the future of my dependents and beneficiaries.

7) I need to work on getting the following documentation in place:

8) I will create a short and long-term budget by this date:

CHAPTER 21
Shifts in the Inner Circle

What greater thing is there for human souls than to feel that they are joined for life – to be with each other in silent unspeakable memories.
~ George Eliot

The diagnosis of a chronic or critical illness changes many things. Next to an impact on physical ability and possibly independence, the impact on personal relationship is perhaps the most profound. Be it a spouse or partner, children, extended family, or with friends, when you get a diagnosis, things tend to shift with your relationships. Sometimes the shifts are subtle, and other times they can feel seismic. Most importantly, you are going to have to learn new ways of interacting with many people in your life, and this can take a brand new set of skills, and some require really open and honest communication.

Romantic Relationships

Dating: Let's start with the pre-cursor to a long-term relationship, the dating game. Starting a new relationship when you also have a diagnosis can be doubly tricky. I was already long-married at the time of my diagnosis, so I don't have any real experience in this arena, but I've watched many friends go through it and seen some really challenging and also some really great things come from their stories.

It seems the ongoing theme is always that when the right person comes along then you'll know it. In addition, anyone who can't handle you, illness and all, isn't good enough for you anyway. I have a feeling these ideas are right. I also have a feeling they can be sort of challenging to wade through while you're in the middle of it. Dating is pretty tricky on its own. Navigating it as a patient can be doubly so.

But it absolutely can be done!! I know lots of chronically ill patients who have found wonderful people to date, and even more wonderful people to marry. People who accept everything about their journey and become an integral piece of it… the other half of it, even. These stories are so heart warming, such as one long-term patient Dorothy Roberts shares:

My husband asked me to marry him, despite my illnesses. However, far from congratulating us, my late mother took him to one side and asked him if he realized what he would be taking on. She explained that our life together would be short as I'd already outlived the medical professions' expectations. Thankfully, he wasn't put off by this, and we have been married for forty one years!!! Life hasn't been easy by any stretch of the imagination. It has often been filled with illness, sadness and pain, but I'm still here and hope that my little story will give hope and encouragement to others.[lxviii]

Your Spouse or Partner: Whether you've taken vows of "in sickness and in health", have a life commitment, or been dating for a while, the onset of a major diagnosis adds a significant aspect to your relationship with your partner. While it's hard to nail down an exact reference to a study, the often-quoted statistics put the divorce rate of couples where at least one partner becomes chronically ill at 75%.

I find this number staggering. But I also get it. Marriage is hard in the best of scenarios. Nobody should be promising otherwise. Add in all the stressors and changes that come when battling a complex set of health problems, and the dynamics in the relationship simply *have to* shift.

My husband and I certainly experienced that. There was a time shortly after our diagnosis where things were incredibly rocky. We fought a lot, over nothing particularly solid. It was just a feeling of disconnect and complex frustrations as we both dealt with my diagnosis in very different ways.

I'm a talker (surprise!), and he is not. I wanted nothing more than to be asked how I was doing, but I didn't want my problems "solved". To this day, he wants to DO things, to fix things. This dynamic would play out in ways that didn't jive very well. I would go to a long doctor's appointment and all I would want is for him to come home and ask me how it went. He would come home knowing it had been a long day for me, and head straight for the dishwasher to empty it. I would be furious because I didn't care about the damn dishes, I cared that my heart and lungs were broken, and he wasn't asking how that all was going. I was looking for emotional support, he was providing help in more concrete ways.

We had to learn to relate to one another by playing to our strengths and re-learning to understand one another's needs. It didn't really matter that we had already been married for about seven years, the old ways of interacting that we thought we knew simply didn't apply any more. I had to learn that as much as it pained me to just come out and ask (falsely thinking he should have known to do so, darn it!), I had to tell him directly the kind of support I needed. I also had to learn to see the kind of support he *was* offering on his own as his unique way of going about things, and that needed to be okay too. He needed to learn to open up and talk about how he felt about my diagnosis and, as hard as it was for him, to take time out of his *doing* to just be there for me. That's a lot of change to ask from both of us, and it doesn't always work perfectly, but we have gotten remarkably better at it over time.

The moral of the story here is that you are going to need to be very open with your partner about how your diagnosis is affecting you. You're also going to need to listen to how your diagnosis is affecting your partner. You're going to have to learn to meet in the middle in new ways, to give one another space to process and grow, but also work together to find new common ground. Like everything else, it is an ongoing process.

There are a few major areas you'll need to work on as a couple that may require some big changes. The more pro-active you can be about talking through these things together and making a plan, the more smooth the sailing can be.

Finances: Does your family need to re-work the budget? Is the healthy spouse going to need to work longer hours or an extra job –

and what affect will that have on the marriage? Can the spouse with the diagnosis find ways to contribute to the family financially if they can no longer work in the job they once did? What sort of outside help might you need to tap into?

Roles at Home: Most couples settle into some sort of routine with keeping up with the house. From shopping, to cooking and cleaning, to taking out the trash, or mowing the lawn, there are probably some consistent jobs you have had and some your partner has probably taken on. These rolls may have to change as your physical abilities change.

One thing that can be a bit of an adjustment is if the rolls have been more traditionally split by gender. In other words, the woman doing the cooking and cleaning, and the man doing the yard work and such. I know not all couples fall into these gender-specific rolls, but many still do. To switch them up can mean more than one partner just taking on more work, or another letting go of some things they used to do. It can really get at the heart of how you identify yourself and your roll in the relationship, and that can be challenging. Continue to be open and honest with one another if any of this comes into play.

Medical Support: Everyone has their own preference regarding how they want their partner to support their medical journey. Some want them by their side at all times, some prefer they show up just for the big stuff. Consider at least having your partner come during the appointments right around the diagnosis, and at any time there is going to be a big shift in approach. You're going to want a second set of ears to hear everything clearly and a person who will ask the questions you forget to. Further, the more your partner understands your course of medical treatment, hopefully the more they'll be able to support you in appropriate ways.

Intimacy: A chronic illness can impact life in the bedroom in some pretty serious ways. Between symptoms, medication side effects, a lack of feeling "sexy" because you really feel like crap, body changes such as medically-related weight gain, fatigue, stress, and so on, it is quite common for the libido of the person being diagnosed to change. Likewise, the healthy partner may have some real concerns about hurting you or risking making something with your health worse.

You really need to be proactive on this front as it can impact the health of a marriage quickly. I can't say it enough – be open and honest with one another. You may want to consult with the doctor on any necessary limitations to begin with. But after that, work together. You may need to find new ways to be intimate, either sexually or emotionally. Finding new ways to connect will help you both maintain some normalcy as well as attend to this very real human need. Handle this part of your relationship with care.

A Very Important Side Note: If you find yourself in a toxic relationship that is not serving you emotionally, or is impacting your health, please consider getting help or getting out. Abuse, be it physical, mental, or emotional is real and is unacceptable. Don't stay in a situation that can hurt you or others (especially children) in your home. It may seem nearly impossible at first, but you can get help and you can get out. I have witnessed some pretty severe controlling or abusive behavior from a healthy partner that is leveled at the one who is sick. That kind of behavior is cowardly and detrimental, and you deserve better.

Your Social Life – Friends and Extended Family

Throughout the course of a diagnosis, the hope is of course that your friends stay near and dear. But the truth is, like in all other areas, there may be some adjustments here too.

There's a fine line between keeping people honestly informed about your illness but not overwhelming them. After all, you live and breathe this thing every day (although hopefully by this far in the book, you've found some great ways to help you work with that!), but your friends and family do not.

It can be easy to lament, *"They just don't understand!"* If you feel that way, you're absolutely right. They don't. Try to re-frame it though. You wouldn't want them to understand the hard parts, right?

The more challenging parts that you have to fight you might not wish on your worst enemy. So on one hand we want empathy and on the other hand, we hope our friends and loved ones never have to know the path we know. Quite the conundrum, isn't it?

Of course, you should be honest when you are asked how you are, and honest when you need some support. That's what the good friends and family are for! But it may also help to sometimes keep it sort of neutral, *"Oh, I have good days and bad..."* and then let them ask for more. Or, you might set up a health journal or blog where you post updates and people can subscribe so they get them. This approach can also be immensely helpful when you are going through something big so that you don't have to update too many individuals at once. Instead, it all gets blasted out to many people at once. Some hospitals provide journal areas, or check out **www.CaringBridge.com**.

You can also set up a simple blog on a site like Blogger or Wordpress. I've done that for a friend and created it to look something like a website. From there she could update us on her progress and I was also able to manage a meal train for her so friends could bring meals specific to her dietary needs (and her kids' preferences!) whenever she was undergoing treatment. This is really quite simple to do and proved to be immensely helpful.

Pick a couple of friends you know you can count on to be your shoulder to cry on, or to lean on, as needed. You might also want to pick one to kick you in the rear as needed. The things we go through as patients of chronic and critical illness are really tough, no doubt. But as we have discussed, it can be a little too easy to slip into very negative thought patterns, or to stay there too long. It's not a bad idea to ask a trusted friend to call you out when you're heading too far in the wrong direction! We all need a little reality check now and then, and this friend can either shake you out of it, or gently tell you it is time to get some help, whichever is needed.

Unfortunately, the time may come when you find you loose some people you were once close to because your illness prevents you from doing the things with them you once were able to. This is a really hard thing to go through! If they left of their own accord, because they just couldn't handle your illness, well, deep shame on them. It may not make it hurt you less, but it is very much their issue. Try to remember that.

On the other hand, if you are finding you can no longer keep up with activities you once enjoyed with your friends, make some really concentrated effort to find new ways to spend time together. Keep that responsibility on you – don't expect them to understand well enough to just make a switch. Grab a cup of tea, ask them over for a cheesy movie night, or enjoy a quiet night of take-out and laughter together. Find new ways to connect with the ones that make you smile, and make sure you're still doing things that make them smile too!

Some people really struggle with their support system after a diagnosis. A feeling of isolation, and sometimes even abandonment, is not uncommon. If that's the case for you, you have a challenge, but it is not one you can't overcome.

Your challenge is to *create* your own new support system. A little later in this book you will read about support groups, both in person and on-line, and those are great places to start. Also consider community resources where you may meet some new people. Churches, local club organizations, and volunteer opportunities are all options. These don't have to be huge undertakings – just what you think you can manage. But an hour or two here or there where you seek the company of others and find something to do together can be invaluable to your sense of self and to your sense of community.

Defining Moment

Take a few minutes to assess one of the important relationships in your life. Who is really special to you that you hope to stay connected with even though a diagnosis may change things? How can you make sure that happens? If your hope is to find a significant other and you'd like to focus on that, use this section to work on how you would connect with your ideal person.

1) The person whose relationship with me I want to focus on is:

2) The way we have interacted in the past includes:

3) I think these are the types of things I should be sharing with them about my everyday experiences with my diagnosis:

(continued on next page)

4) Here are three ways we can still have an amazing time together, even if I'm not feeling up to our old activities

a.

b.

c.

Chapter 22
The Questions With Kids

The attitude that you have as a parent is what your kids will learn from, more than what you tell them. They don't remember what you try to teach them. They remember what you are.
~Jim Henson

Family Planning

If you are in your childbearing years, sometimes you are faced with the incredibly difficult decision on whether or not to have a child – either your first, or an additional one. Sometimes, that choice is made for you, and there are few things that rock someone who desires to be a parent more than hearing that maybe you can't be one.

If traditional childbirth is not an option for you because of your health, there are still choices. They aren't always easy – you may have to grapple with tough questions around your ability to raise a child with your illness, but know that many people certainly find a way. You may need to go through a long process of paperwork, interviews, and waiting to adopt and that can demand significant emotional and financial resources.

Also be sure to consider not only potential physical stress of keeping up after a young child, but the financial changes you'll need to be prepared for as well. Once you've decided to grow your family, but know that you aren't going to be doing it the old fashioned way, new decisions must be made. This is the hard part, but it can also be the fun part because, ideally, at the end of it you have your little one. Keep your eye on that prize!

Surrogacy is one path some people choose to take. Jessie Kohler generously shared this experience:

When I was diagnosed with Pulmonary Arterial Hypertension in 2004, my now-husband and I quickly learned that it would be unlikely that I could safely carry a child to term without risking my life and the life of the baby. After waiting for my medical condition to stabilize, we spent several years considering various ways of becoming parents, including adoption. After much thought and discussion, we chose to pursue surrogacy because we really wanted to experience the joy of creating a life ourselves from the very beginning and being there during the pregnancy and birth of our child.

We found a wonderful surrogate through an agency who wanted to be matched with parents who would be involved in the process. She and her family (husband and three girls) quickly became like family. We exchanged frequent calls, attended ultrasound appointments via Facetime and in person and were able to attend the birth of our daughter in Wisconsin despite the fact that she was a month early! I was the first person to hold our daughter and my husband cut her umbilical cord. We continue to be close to our surrogate and her family today.

There are challenges in the surrogacy process, however. It can be very expensive, especially if you are going through an agency. Some families minimize these costs by finding a surrogate among friends or family who agree to carry without a fee. For someone with PH, it can also be challenging if you want to use your own eggs – hormones must be injected and eggs retrieved under general anesthesia although another alternative is to use an egg donor. It was sometimes hard during the process to not be experiencing the pregnancy myself, but we felt so blessed to have the option of surrogacy, a wonderful surrogate to carry our child, and a healthy baby that those thoughts were fleeting. Today we are the parents of a beautiful daughter who brings us so much joy and hope.[lxix]

If surrogacy is not for you, adoption in this country remains a real and also very much needed (for the child and the parent!) option. Adoption options vary widely from state to state, so you'll need to do some research on what's allowed where you live. Expect that you can consider private adoption through an agency or maybe a private lawyer, domestic and international children, and also adoption through the social services system where you would consider taking a foster child.

When the time came to expand our family, our story took a very long time to come about. I was ready quite a bit before my husband, and we had to learn a very new way of working together as we made this decision, just like we have learned new ways of relating in so many other areas. Ultimately though, we are preparing to adopt a little girl through the foster system. As I've shared this part of my journey with other patients, I found it has resonated very deeply, and so I would like to share it with you as well.

My journey to her began at age 19. It was the year I took the job as a nanny for a little girl newly adopted from China. I clearly remember rocking her to sleep in my arms, gazing down at that gorgeous perfect little face, and having the wind sucked out of me. What if her parents had not cared enough to go and get her? What if she had stayed in a Chinese orphanage? What hell of a life would she have lived? And here she was, safe in their home, safe in my arms, the world at her feet. I vowed then that I too would make the difference in a little life, and adopt.

I knew the child I got would be a girl... Altruistically speaking, girls have a pretty tough time in much of the world and I wanted to make a difference for one. Totally selfishly perhaps, I wanted to raise a ballet dancer, like me, someone to share that with (for as long as she would tolerate it before asserting independence, of course!).

Eight years ago I had another brush with adoption that only further solidified these feelings. I was teaching special education and I had twin girls from India on my case load. They were the result of a botched late-term abortion and had survived, eventually being adopted by an American couple. Again, I found myself looking at them and thinking, "What if..."

Fast forward many years, and I have an incredible biological son. A son who is my own miracle - as we now know I shouldn't have survived the pregnancy because I probably had PH already, and we just didn't know it.

When you have PH you can't get pregnant. Or, at least, you really shouldn't. This is something you're told pretty much upon diagnosis. When I was told, it didn't faze me. My son was an infant at the time, and pregnancy was not something I was too big of a fan of the first time around. Since I already knew I wanted to adopt, I figured that would be our route, and that was totally cool.

Except, for a long time it wasn't our route at all. I was so busy chasing a toddler and trying to get better and trying to be self-employed, and my husband always works so hard, and our lives were just full. Although we batted the idea of adoption around many times, the answer always seemed to be "Not now." And that was fine.

But then a little over a year ago my damn biological clock started ticking...and chiming... and the gong started going off... and I couldn't make it stop. I wanted that baby.

After long heart-to-hearts with my husband, it was clear he just wasn't ready for adoption. And I couldn't blame him. It's not like other times when we've disagreed and my nose is all out of joint because he doesn't see it my way (come on, you know you all get like that). This time, he had real fears about the future. How the financial burden of supporting our family is by and large on him. And worse, he had fears about being a single parent some day, if PH took the ultimate toll. These aren't fears we face head on too often. In fact, we never had before. We've chosen to live with the positive and not think that way. But when we're choosing to discuss a very purposeful choice for the long-term future, and involve the life of a child, we kind of have to wrestle with that dark side too.

For the sake of my marriage, I vowed to force this clock away. MAKE it go away. Focus on my son - whom I love and adore and is so so so enough in all possible ways. Basically, I tried to beat my biology. And pretend I was winning. And I did okay... for a while.

Then in the spring of 2013 I attended a dance recital. And I sat there and looked at the moms around me smiling with so much pride for their daughters on stage and I just lost it. I sat in the dark auditorium and cried silently. That should have been me. PH robbed that from me.

The grief followed me in the months ahead, although I tried to keep it in. Baby showers were torture. My sister got pregnant and I cried my way through shopping for the niece whose arrival I was over the moon excited for. And finally it was clear that I was going to have to either get some serious professional help in letting this all go, or re-visit the decision.

I tentatively broached the topic with my husband. And... he said yes. Why the timing is right now, I just don't know (neither does he). But my health is stable (thriving, even), all of my doctors are 100% in support of this decision, my business is growing, things have changed... and now we're ready as a couple and as a family.

Then it was just down to deciding on how to get her. International adoption held little draw now. I wasn't that interested in having to travel overseas with PH to go and collect her. Domestic adoption sure sounded good, but the tens of thousands of dollars it costs seriously deterred us. Surrogacy was also on the table... but I ended up deciding that if we really were going to do this, I needed to stay true to my original intent all those years ago and help a child in need.

And so, we were left with the foster system. We have chosen to adopt through social services and take a child whose parents cannot care for her. It does not escape me that for us to get our daughter, someone else will lose theirs. Realizing this fact humanizes the birth parents, whom I might otherwise have had some pretty big issues with, given that in order for the child to come to us, her birth parents would have to be a danger to her, and I just can't imagine who would hurt a child.

This path is scary. In fact, I should probably be much more jittery about it than I am. Our daughter may come to us drug exposed, abused, neglected... who knows. We could be placed with a child, only to have the arrangement fall through because the system deems reunification with the birth family or extended family is better. But the truth is, the road to her has been so very long, sometimes so very hard, and now is the time.

It is going to be fine.

I have total peace about it. A peace that surpasses understanding, and I'm pretty content with that. All of our state licensure requirements are complete. Now, all we have to do is wait for her.

Caring for Children

When you've received a significant diagnosis and there are children, or hopes for children, in the mix, things can seem infinitely complicated. If you are already a parent, you may need to learn to relate to your children in different ways than you have previously, or how you imagined it would be. The following guidelines were originally co-written by me and published by the Pulmonary Hypertension Association[lxx].

Depending on the age of the child(ren) in question, your needs in how you care for them may vary. Don't be afraid to ask for help. If your physical functioning has been impacted by your diagnosis, look for new ways to interact together. Low-key activities such a board games, reading a good book together, or going on special outings where you can sit as needed are wonderful ways to spend time.

As with so many other things, you may need to get creative on how you approach this part of your life. You may need to ask for help with childcare or carpooling (or you might be perfect for carpooling because driving is sitting!).

I know it can be incredibly hard to think about not giving our kids the life we think we should, the life you as a parent without a major diagnosis might have provided. We want the world for our kids. But kids are remarkably resilient. Given the right tools and expectations, they can also be remarkably compassionate and certainly a help as they get older. There may need to be shifts in activities and mindset that may need to happen. They may not be easy sometimes. But there are always choices.

If you have a serious diagnosis and you are a parent, talking to your children about your illness may be one of the most challenging emotional issues you will face with this disease. Even if you are a relative such as an aunt, uncle, or a grandmother, talking about your diagnosis with the little ones in your life can be a tough conversation, and one that must be taken on very mindfully.

What follows is meant to serve only as a general guide to begin this important conversation. It is highly recommended that after you read this section that you take the next step of consulting with child development experts who know your child and your family personally, such as your pediatrician and a teacher or school guidance counselor.

To begin with, what you tell your children hinges very much on age and developmental level. The things a pre-schooler is ready to hear will vary from those that an elementary student can handle, and a teenager will need more still. Use these age guidelines to help plan and inform your conversations. In addition, since how your disease affects you will most likely change over time, what information you give your children may need to change over time as well.

Infants and Toddlers: Even if you aren't saying much at home during the diagnosis period or about your current treatments, be aware that even at this young age children may be aware that something is amiss. Be prepared for the possibility of changes in your very young child's behavior, such as disruptions in sleep patterns, regression of milestones (such as potty training), and increased behavioral issues such as tantrums or aggression. These are ways that very small children let us know that they are aware something is different in their world, even when they cannot understand or express it. Stay calm, stick to your routine, and be as nurturing and patient as possible. Remember, when it comes to a baby or toddler's behavior, most often "this too shall pass."

Quick Tips (Ages 0-3)

- Keep to normal routine, as much as possible. Familiar surroundings and consistency mean security.
- Use a normal voice and maintain composure to reassure a toddler.
- Any changes in routine should be explained to the child in terms of how it will affect them personally. This explanation should come prior to the change if possible. For example, *"Mommy feels bad today and needs to take a nap, so she can't play with you right now."*
- Give lots of love and attention. Don't stop, even if they seem inconsolable. Hugs are wonderfully reassuring to small children.

Pre-schoolers: Preschoolers are self-centered, concrete thinkers. Children at this age may ask questions about your oxygen or medication supplies that they can see, but the inner workings of the diagnosis you have will be well beyond them. Be honest, but don't give any more information than the child needs to know or wants to ask. Simple answers like, *"That is Mommy's medicine."* or *"That helps Daddy breathe well at night."* will most likely suffice small curiosity. If, however, you have a *"But WHY???"* stage on your hands, continue to stick to simple answers: *"Because the doctor says it helps."* Or, *"Because we do things to keep our bodies healthy and this is one thing I do."* etc.

If there is a chance you could become too ill to care for your pre-schooler for a while, or may have to go to the hospital for a stay, children at this age want to know one thing: *"Who will take care of me?"*

Don't take it personally if they aren't overly concerned about your own well-being at that moment – that's not how their little minds are wired to work just yet. Think through this question ahead of time and come up with a list of special people who will be there for your child if this kind of situation arises. Share the list of people with other caregivers and teachers so that your child can receive a consistent message. Children at this age thrive on predictability, sense of security, and routine. In so much as it is possible, make sure these things are in place in case of a crisis.

Another thing to be aware of is that children in preschool may process their understanding of your illness through play. They may act out "doctor" with more sophistication than their peers if they are aware of things like medication pumps, wheelchairs, and nasal cannulas. While this may be a bit unsettling for you, understand that it is a child's natural way of processing and exploring information. Any fear or uncertainty they have may also be displayed in their play, so be on the lookout for signs that your child is worried about your illness and don't hesitate to contact your pediatrician for advice on how to best support them at this stage.

Quick Tips (Ages 3-5)
- Small children need lots of hugs when there is an illness/disease in the family. They need extra love and attention and reassurance that they will be cared for.
- Matter-of-fact and brief answers to questions are important. Your feelings should be shared in a simplified manner. For example, *"I miss Daddy,"* or *"I hurt inside."*
- Encourage physical activity, drawing, and music to help the child express their own emotions.
- If the parent is hospitalized, it helps to keep a few of the child's toys and books at the hospital so they have something familiar to play with when they visit.

Elementary Age: Children at this age are still concrete thinkers, but they are able to visualize on a more abstract level as well. You may want to use a doll or a bear to show where the parts of the body impacted by your diagnosis are so that they can see thing in a way, which matches their concrete way of processing the universe at this age. Again, as with younger children, keep your conversations brief and at a basic level. Answer questions very honestly, but don't provide more information than the child asks or can handle.

You may need to be prepared for questions about your mortality (*"Are you going to die?"*), if the disease is contagious (*"Can I catch it?"*) and feelings of guilt (*"Did Mommy get sick because I was naughty?"*). Think through how you will answer these questions for your child. If they aren't asked, don't raise them on your own.

If you are at a critical state and realize you have to have a very difficult decision about your passing, take some time to prepare and to build a network of support – both for you and your child. When you do have the conversation, be honest by explaining that all living things will some day pass away, but try not to focus on the fact that your passing may be sooner than a healthy parent's (remember, we don't know when medication is going to turn things around or a cure will be found!).

Children at this age still may not react to your illness in a way you might expect. Even after you tell them you are sick, they may run off and play as usual. Do not take this personally! They may need time to process, or they may not have fully grasped the idea just yet. They will process things in time, and may come to you later with more questions or fears that need to be discussed.

As with pre-schoolers, look for changes in behavior that signal your child is having difficulty understanding or coping. Depending on how you feel about sharing information on your illness, talking to school personnel may be a very good idea. Classroom teachers appreciate this kind of information so that they can be sensitive to your child's needs during the day. School counselors may be available to help your child process feelings. Taking a team approach with the school may be the best way to support your child.

Quick Tips (Ages 5-9)
- Early school age children need gentle honesty. If they don't receive clear explanations about what is happening with their parent's illness or treatment, they will make sense of it by using their imagination and incorrect information.
- Ask children frequently if they have any questions. They may need many invitations to talk before they feel comfortable voicing a concern. If kids aren't ready to talk, that's okay too.

- Ask the child to explain back to you what is happening to the parent who is sick. This will help you know what they comprehend and help you correct any misconceptions the child may have.
- Reassure children they will be cared for and that it is normal to feel angry or afraid.
- Show your feelings to encourage them to share theirs. A sad movie, story or song can encourage reluctant children to express their feelings.
- Unless the child asks for more time with a parent in the hospital, keep hospital visits brief.

Quick Tips (Ages 9-12)
- Children at this age can assume additional responsibilities but they shouldn't be overloaded. Don't let the child assume the role of either parent.
- Preteens might seem "selfish" about the way the illness affects them. Try to be patient with them. Instead of punishing children, talk with them.
- Show affection.
- Model ways for children to deal with feelings and worries.
- Preteens want specific information about prognosis and treatment. Answer their questions and promise them more information as it becomes available.
- Many children will use the Internet to find more information. This can be scary if the information is negative or too technical. Be aware of where they are gathering their information.
- Offer to talk to their friends and their friends' parents to explain what is happening.
- Keep appropriate people at your child's school informed about your situation so they can help you with any behavior changes that occur.

Adolescents and Teenagers: By adolescence, kids are able to understand significantly more. The best approach at this age is complete openness and honesty. As with children of younger ages, take your cues from them and don't over-share.

It is okay to ask more leading questions at this stage to encourage conversation from a teen who may be a reluctant communicator or who is afraid to upset you. Remember we live in the age of the Internet, so if you don't talk about it, the computer very well might! Be sure you are steering your teen to the right information.

Because they are better able to understand and talk about your condition, it could be tempting to lean on your child as your primary source of emotional support, but this is probably not the best approach. This is not to say that you shouldn't talk about your feelings together, but avoid asking your teenager to assume an adult role. Keep the lines of communication open and balanced.

Ask your child if they want to talk to a counselor or another trusted adult about their feelings. Know that teenagers' friends are central in their worlds right now and they may choose to lean on them instead of you. Sharing with your teen's friends' parents may help so that other adults can be ready to offer assistance and guidance if necessary.

Quick Tips (Ages 13-18)
- Because people outside the family are so important to them, teens usually cope better than younger children with a seriously ill parent.
- Be aware that teens are feeling torn between a desire to be with their friends and with their sick parent.
- Encourage them to keep up with as many normal social activities as possible.
- Friends are an important source of support for teens.
- Avoid making your teen assume adult roles but involve them in some decision-making activities, too.
- Offer to talk to their friends and their friends' parents to explain what is happening.

In Conclusion: Remember that above all, with children of any age, reassure your child that you love them unconditionally and that getting sick is something that happens sometimes, even when we don't really understand why. Also reassure them it is not their fault that their parent is sick.

If your family has a faith or spirituality you wish to impart to your children, be sure to weave that into these difficult conversations. Offer your child an open line of communication. Be on the lookout for signs that they need extra support, and use your community resources as much as necessary.

Defining Moment

Take some time to think about the kids in your world. They may be your own children, the children of family members (nieces and nephews, grandchildren, etc.), or kids in the neighborhood. If they are going to be impacted somehow by your diagnosis, take some time to think about how you can plan to support them.

1) The kids in my world are (names and ages):

2) The questions they might have about my diagnosis right now are:

(continued on next page)

3) The questions they might have later on (as they get older or as your condition changes) are:

4) I can address their concerns by using these words and explanations *(If the children belong to someone else, please speak to their parents prior to having a conversation, if at all possible.)*:

CHAPTER 23
A Hand Up

There's a certain grace in accepting what your life is and embracing all the good things that have been – but there's still an expectation of good things to come. Not necessarily what you expected.
~Emmylou Harris

Even with the intensity of medical tests, the regime of medications, and the back and forth to what can seem like countless doctor's appointments, perhaps one of the most unexpected aspects of a diagnosis has little to do with these external factors, and more to do with the internal response they demand.

Combining the halting or re-writing of life's plans, and the uncertainty of the future, a diagnosis can send you careening off the course you thought you lived on. When it comes right down to it though, it is the loss of autonomy that can really take the biggest toll.

Do you hate asking for help? If so, you are not alone! It can be very challenging to transition from a life of independence to needing to rely on people for things that once came easy to you. Things as simple as grocery shopping, or as complex as your finances, whatever it is, it's sometimes the hardest pill to swallow. By my observation and experience, there are a few primary reasons patients tend to balk at asking for help.

You don't want to look weak: Our culture carries a very strong sense of individuality. It can feel counter-intuitive to admit you need help or ask for a favor, especially when we've been somewhat programmed to be the ones who "do it all".

You don't want to impose on friends and family: An extension of the sense of individuality is the idea people put on themselves that if you *do* ask for help, you are somehow a burden, or are imposing.

You don't want to admit your own limitations – to yourself or others: It can be really hard on the ego to admit you need help, especially if you've enjoyed a certain sense of autonomy in the past.

It can be equally difficult to show that vulnerability to others.

You don't want to face that the answer to your request for help might in fact have to be a "no", or "not right now": Even if you can get to the place where you might be okay asking for help, the answer may not be the one you were looking for. And then you fear facing any disappointment or embarrassment that could follow.

I get each of these reasons. I've seen them play out, and being quite independent (and stubborn), I've lived a fair number of them. But the truth is, a major diagnosis changes things (you knew that), and so, like everything else with this "new normal", you'll have to adjust. You have a choice, and that choice rests on your internal reaction to the external factor that you need help with. In other words, when you enter an interaction, you also have power over your reaction. This means you also guide the outcome, because much of the outcome is based on how you perceive the situation as it plays out. This power you have leaves you with a few basic choices.

You can skip asking for the help at all: Before you do this, consider the cost – your pride may be intact, but what about your health? It can be really hard to let go of some of that ego, I know. But if you don't, and your health suffers, is it worth it?

You can ask for help, but resent what is given to you: This is perhaps the trickiest place to be. You're resentful of the fact you even need help to begin with, but then being unsatisfied with the help you do receive compounds that. Perhaps this is because the person helping you isn't doing it "your way".

Try to see the help under a different paradigm: Those reaching out to support you want to help *you*, of course, but it may also be their own way of fighting back too. It's pretty painful to watch a friend or loved one suffer under disease. Most friends and family lack the medical expertise to swoop in and offer effective treatment or a cure, but that doesn't lessen their desire to do *something*. And that feeling of helplessness as a loved one suffers is awful.

If power and control over how things are done is your challenge, it's time to adjust again. Most likely, you really do need to learn to let a little of that control go! Take a minute for an honest check-in with yourself. Do you *really* need to fuss when the laundry isn't folded your way, or the brand of cereal brought home isn't the brand you usually buy? Probably not.

But what if whatever about the help is bothering you really is a sticking point for you, and you just can't settle over what is being done? In that case, it's time for an honest, gentle, adult conversation with your helper. It's okay to stand your ground when you need to as well. It's about a balance between your reaction and expectations, and where your true needs are.

So, if you need to address how something is being done when someone is helping you out, first sit down with your helper for an honest and pro-active conversation.. First, thank them most sincerely for the help they are giving. And then quietly and calmly explain what your sticking point is… what you need changed, and why. Ask them how you can support them within your capabilities.

For instance, my husband needs the most detailed shopping list ever, and then he needs to call me from the grocery store… three times. And it drives me crazy. And I have to be okay with it if I want the help! So I support him helping me by making the list and answering the phone all three times. It's not perfect, but it's our dynamic and it works.

Whatever the outcome, thank them again for their help. Cranky recipients of help may find themselves otherwise quite alone if a little care isn't taken in the approach.

Or, you can accept the help gladly, and look for ways to pay it forward in other areas of your life. Imagine a universe where the recipient of any good will reaches out to another further down the road and passes on the blessing. What a beautiful world we could create.

In the end, try to see their help as their hand in your battle. As one patient, Patty Farrow told me, "*I know how good I feel when I'm able to help someone but it took me a while to realize that I had the ability to help others feel the same. Sometimes the help they give isn't even about you...it's about them,* "[lxxi]

It is a good thing to say you need help, it is perhaps an even braver thing to accept it. I know it isn't easy. Our pride gets in the way. Our desire to do it all tries to drown out our body's call for help. Maybe, just maybe, we don't want to admit to ourselves our own new and necessary boundaries. Re-framing this experience so you see it as a positive interaction between you and those who love you will be priceless. After all, you know you'd do the same for them.

I've been through this even with people in my world who become sick. As they start to falter, I want to fight harder, and more and more on their behalf. And I just can't do much about where they are in their medical journey. I can't fix the medication problems, or calm the storm at the hospital. But I can fix a meal, send a gift card, or even a note of support online. And for heaven's sake, if that's all I can do, then that's what I want to do. Let others do the same for you. And let a little of their grace and strength carry you for a bit. You can pay it forward later. No matter what form of support you choose, do not experience this alone.

Defining Moment

Take some time to get honest with yourself about the help you need, the help you ask for, and the way you allow yourself to think about that help.

1) What kind of help do I need now? *This may be concrete, like with shopping or cleaning, or it could be more abstract, such as asking for prayer or needing a good friend to let you vent.*

2) How do I go about asking for help when I need it? How do I feel about my approach?

3) How do I go about accepting help when it is offered? How do I feel about my reaction?

(continued on next page)

4) Is there anything I really need to say to my helpers to make our time together and their gift of help to me more effective or comfortable?

5) What, if any, adjustments can I make to my view of accepting help gracefully so that I can spend time and energy focusing on being well and devoting the time and energy you have to self-care or the things in life that matter most to me?

CHAPTER 24
Finding Your Second Family

The "I" in illness is isolation, and the crucial letters in wellness are we.
~Author unknown

Throughout this journey you are on, the greatest gift you can give is to be there for others. You'll get it back ten-fold in return too. Banding together is not always easy. For starters, I know a lot of people who don't go to support groups because they don't want to be around people whose disease has progressed further than their own. This is a pretty reasonable concern. It can feel incredibly vulnerable to reach out and make a friend who shares your disease when you know the tough truth is that they may suffer in front of you and perhaps even pass away. But there is so much inherent value to these groups too.

It seems living with a chronic or critical illness can be a constant series of one-two punches. A great appointment? Flying! A bad one... seismic crash. An incredible time connecting with other people who really get you? Fly. Another patient you've grown to care for passes? Seismic crash. A dear friend in dire health straights... and you freeze, just waiting and praying for it to be okay. And the events always seem to come one after the next. Up. Down. Fly. Crash.

It's really hard to watch the world spin sometimes. Bad things happen to good people, those we care about have to carry burdens we wish we could shoulder for them. Sometimes hard times seem to have no answer to the question, "Why?"

A few years ago I sat in a funeral for a baby girl, the daughter of a friend. There was absolutely nothing in that moment that could have been said to me to bring peace or make the situation okay, at least I didn't think so. Because, really, how do you justify suffering and tragedy?

Well, the priest somehow managed to find just the right words. He spoke of our tears that day, how they were blessed. He said we have a choice in life. We can open our hearts and love, and risk our hearts being broken. Or, we can keep our hearts closed, and the price for that is a shriveled and cold heart. Each of us sat there that day totally broken-hearted, the tears flowing. And yet, it was because of the choice we had made to love the family who was saying goodbye to their baby girl. And so, because we opened our hearts, those tears were blessed. We had done the right thing, as painful as it was.

In that moment, I did feel peace. The pain of what I was witnessing didn't leave, but somehow, somehow... it was going to be okay, because in the human experience, here we were with open and broken hearts, loving someone who needed it.

I could not help but to relate all this to having a critical illness too. Being so involved in my disease community means I see and experience a lot of heartbreak. A lot. More than I feel like I can handle sometimes. And yet, I've chosen to open my heart. And if I have to be here, it is a blessed place to be. To make a difference. To have people coming into my life and change it in ways I wouldn't have imagined. I never knew I could so unconditionally love people I had never met, or only spent a handful of hours with, and yet... here we are.

Support group leader Doug Taylor puts the value of patient-to-patient support beautifully,

Most people when diagnosed with a rare disease have never heard of it before. Even if they have heard of it, they probably have never met anyone who has it. Thus, the diagnosis brings confusion as well as a feeling of isolation.

Support groups can break that isolation by introducing newly diagnosed patients to others who share their diagnosis. Support groups offer a safe environment for people to ask questions without having to worry that they are going to be laughed at.

Support groups, or rather the people who attend support groups, can be a great source of information. Often, when our doctors tell us things, the information goes over our heads. Members of support groups can help a new patient understand some of that information. Members can help new patients come up with the right questions to ask their healthcare team.

Support groups are also a great resource for finding the right doctor to treat you. Members can share their experiences with doctors as well as their experiences with particular medications.

People often hear the term "support group" and get the impression that it is a bunch of people sitting around complaining and crying. Nothing could be further from the truth, at least for the support group meetings I've attended. If someone does get emotional, it is OK. There are friends there to share their grief or fears and offer them encouragement. But most of the time, the sound of laughter is more common than the sound of tears.[lxxii]

To find a group near you, visit your disease's national association, ask your doctor, or search around online.

Online Groups

If there isn't a support group in your area, or you'd like a different kind of support (24/7 most likely!) try to find a group online. I'll bet if you do a quick Facebook search using the name of your diagnosis you may find an easy dozen.

A little word to the wise with online groups… they can sometimes be tricky to navigate. The Internet itself is a wonderful place, full of opportunities to learn more things and connect with people from around the world who are sharing in your journey, and who can become crucial to your support system.

I learned the power of connecting with fellow patients online very early. First it was on a discussion board provided by the Pulmonary Hypertension Association. I found myself there in some of the earliest days after diagnosis. The people I met became a lifeline.

They helped me learn what to expect from my medication options, could explain to me in ways nobody else could why I was having trouble coping sometimes (because they GOT IT!), assured me I would be okay on the days I felt the least like it was possible, and just generally held me up while I found my footing again after my diagnosis. I would have been lost without them.

While there were really wonderful people I was meeting online, there was also something missing for me. One of the things I was struggling with personally was raising a toddler at the same time I was not doing so well physically. I had a lot of questions about raising a young child while being a patient - and I could not for the life of me find any other young moms who shared my diagnosis. In fact, it took me a solid year to locate one. Too long, for sure.

Besides raising kids, other young adult patients began speaking up about issues they were struggling with that seemed pretty unique to our demographic. The Pulmonary Hypertension Association responded by pulling together a team of four patients, myself included, to create something called Generation Hope, a solely online support system for young adults. We are still going strong today, and have created a community of a couple of hundred patients who work hard to support one another, I am so proud of what we've built and so grateful for the fact that we are there for one another.

As usual, the big things that have happened in my health journey really are quite simple. They come about by figuring out there's a need, either for myself and usually for others like me, and not stopping until I figure out how to get that need met. There's no reason at all you can't rise above what is in your own life and create the same things.

As great as banding online and using the internet can be, being online can be weird and crazy and sometimes, unfortunately, just downright nasty too. In an online support forum, all facets come out, the good, the bad, and the "what the heck are they thinking??"

There's something about a more or less anonymous forum, the kind where you can say things, but not to someone's face, that brings out attributes in people that are less than savory. If the pen is mightier than the sword, then the keyboard is mightier than a land-mine. Words get put out there and can detonate in unexpected ways and places. Intended or not, what we say online is taken in the context constructed by the receiver. They take in this information without the benefit of watching your facial expression or hearing you tone of voice. What it pretty much boils down to is the simple fact that it is incredibly easy for things to be misunderstood.

Unfortunately, I've watched all too often as wonderful groups come to virtual blows, and even implode. I suppose it is bound to happen. As people become an online community, we are in fact creating a sort of organized society. Social rules and agreed upon standards of conduct must emerge (it really helps if they are clearly set from the beginning). Leaders will arise, and some people will find the group culture just isn't a good fit for them. This isn't necessarily a bad thing. We can't all fit in everywhere, and nor should we. What a boring place the world would be.

What should always be the binding factor though is that if you engage in these groups, you are united by one thing, a common disease state that you all would do well to fight together. Keep a civil tongue (or more precisely, keyboard!), and don't engage with the rabble-rousers. As my dad says, *"Never wrestle with pigs. You both get dirty and the pigs love it."*

This simple guideline can help you engage in and even create a community of people that will become some of your dearest friends – even if you never even meet in person! I am often surprised at the bond I feel with my virtual community. I laugh with them, cry with them, and celebrate their successes. When they fall ill, I worry as if they were just down the street, and not half a world away. I know they do the same for me.

What follows is a template that provides guidelines for online groups. I co-wrote it with some of my colleagues at the Pulmonary Hypertension Association and we use it with Generation Hope. [lxxiii]

Terms of Use

The (name of group) was created to give (name of disease) patients who are/have (describe target patient group) a way to receive and give support, as well as, to share information with others. Our desire is that everyone feels welcome and that (name of group) is a safe and supportive place for all involved.

Please remember that all online community participants have something significant in common with you: Their life has been changed by (disease). While we may have many differences, making the best of our lives with (disease) is our common ground.

In addition, please remember that as a part of (name of group), you represent the group to both the (disease) community in general and to the public. We do have ramifications for membership, and strive to maintain a very positive community. While there are many people who will fall into our target community, we ask all participants to be mindful that some of what we discuss may be a sensitive subject for some, not all places are right for all people, and that there are many wonderful groups out there for (disease) patients of all walks of life.

By participating on our forums, you agree to the following:

1.While participants are welcome to share personal experiences with (disease state), nothing posted on these forums should be considered a substitute for medical advice. Please consult with your physician for all health-related decisions.

2. Electronic messages lack the nuances of face-to-face and telephone conversations. When composing a message, please try to be as clear about your intent as possible, as to minimize offending others. When reading a message, please remember that the written word may be open to interpretation.

3. The use of ALL CAPITAL LETTERS in an online post or message is considered yelling and can cause difficulty when reading. Please use words in all capital letters sparingly.

4. Messages with profane language or that contain harmful comments about an individual or group is prohibited and may be removed at a moderator's discretion. See below for details about reporting a problem message.

5. All listed contact information of members, and anything posted by members, should be kept strictly confidential within the group. Further, this information cannot be used for purposes outside of (name of group) (marketing, mailing lists, research, etc.)

Reporting a Problem
Should you have concern about an interaction on our boards, first consider the idea that in online communication misunderstandings can easily happen. You may wish to politely ask for clarification on intended meaning before moving forward.

Should you wish to report a problem, please contact one of our moderators (list them):

We hope the forums meet the needs of the community by providing an easily accessible way to communicate, exchange support and share information any time of any day. We welcome you to our group.

Defining Moment

Do some research and see if there are local support groups in your area. Try asking your doctor or just searching online. Record what you find out.

Support Group Name:

Location of Meeting:

Day and Time:

Next, Do a search for online support systems. Check national organizations for your disease to see what they provide, as well as more informal locations such as Facebook. Record the location and purpose of the top 5 groups you find. Then spend some time exploring each to see which may be a good fit.

Group name	Location (URL)	Notes

CHAPTER 25
I Take My Shoes as Seriously As My Medication

Do your thing and don't care if they like it
~Tina Fey

What does it take to cope with a major diagnosis? Beyond the doctors' visits, the medications, even the things outlined in this book? What does it really take?

It takes being tuned in to what makes you happy, and then knowing you're worth it enough to make those things happen, to chase them down, to practice them regularly, but to especially practice them when you know you're facing a hard time. Find those things and create little rituals for yourself, and tap into them as often as possible.

I realize it may sound trite in the big scheme of things, but shoes make me happy. They just do. From the fact that I am five foot two and a good set of heels makes my pants fit better so I'm not dragging them on the ground, to the fact that a sweet stiletto is just… fun. Shoes make me smile, I feel good in a great pair, and better when I wear ones with a little sass to them than I do in boring old sneakers (although I did just buy purple sneakers, so even those have gotten better).

I was lucky to find my "thing" early on. During the diagnosis process I had to have what is called a VQ scan to check for clots in my lungs. I got it into my head to wear four-inch heel suede boots to that appointment. I was not happy about the tests, but that particular pair of shoes made me happy, so wear them I did… right into the machine.

Since I go to a teaching hospital, it so happened that the person doing the test was a student, and since the machine used was on that you lay on and that moves in all four directions while they scan your lungs, it also turned out that I had the equivalent of a student drive. A bad student driver.

I was jerked around so many times on that machine that I was a bit nauseous by the end of the test. Plus I was actually radioactive from the dye they used, and hence warned that if the police had their scanners out that day, I may be pulled over heading home.

Nauseous, scared, sad, and a possible threat to national security? Not a great day. But the shoes were great, in fact they were the only things that day that *was* great, and I promised myself from then on that I would always wear great shoes to every crappy appointment. And I have.

I have another funny little habit, this one attached to a sweet story. I only take my pills at home from a wine glass. I actually started that one pretty early on too, and somewhere along the way my family caught on. Two years after I was diagnosed, I opened up a Christmas present, and nestled in the box was a beautiful hand-blown cobalt blue wine glass. Tucked into the glass was a check – large enough to send me to my first pulmonary hypertension conference (a conference that would change my life). I ended up going to the conference on a scholarship and used the check instead to fly my brother home from across the country for a visit, but it has been almost five years and I still use that wine glass everyday.

I've talked to a lot of patients about the things that they do to feel better when they're doing something related to their diagnosis. Some of them decorate their medical equipment – the crazier the better. Some plan a special stop at a beach or a favorite restaurant to break up a long drive to a far-off medical facility. Others save a little money each time they go to an appointment and then when it adds up, they buy themselves something special.

The point here really is to tune into the things that bring you joy – even if they seems silly. Then do them regularly. Make sure you laugh a lot along the way. It can be so easy to get overwhelmed in just the everyday management of our lives as patients. There's so much to keep track of, to do, to try to pace yourself through. Go ahead and choose those little indulgences that give you a smile every time you get to do them. It's worth the time you take to lighten the load just a bit.

Defining Moment

What are the little things in life that give you a smile? Brainstorm some nice things you can do for yourself. Try to come up with at least one you can do every day and at least one that is an indulgence, maybe for a "special occasion" or that you can do around a big medical event such as an appointment, test, or the start of a new medication, etc. Then plan to make them happen!

What I plan to do	What I'll need to prepare for so it gets done (buy supplies, save some $$, etc.)	How I will feel when it is in place and I get to enjoy it

CHAPTER 26
Preparing for the Final Chapter

*"What's wrong with death, sir? What are we so mortally afraid of?
Why can't we treat death with a certain amount of humanity and
dignity, and decency, and God forbid, maybe even humor. Death is
not the enemy gentlemen."*
~Robin Williams as Patch Adams

This may be one of the more difficult chapters for some people to read. The hard truth is that we as a culture have a very difficult time addressing issues surrounding death and dying. But for those of us whose illnesses come with a shorter-than-average life expectancy, we are forced to grapple with the topic much earlier than we ever dreamed.

I understand and completely empathize with the fact that this is an uncomfortable topic for many. It's hasn't always been a particularly comfortable topic for me either, although I would wager my take on it is a little bit different than some might expect. I promise not to dwell on the macabre here. So bear with me.

If I am to be totally frank about my own disease, the life expectancy with PH sucks. Completely and utterly sucks. When I was diagnosed in 2008, the life expectancy was about 50% at five years. That's a whole lot to take in, and a lot of acceptance to come to.

All has not turned out as bleak as it might have seemed though. It turns out I continue to defy the odds with every breath I take. New treatments keep hitting the market, and newer data has bumped up average survival to more like seven years[lxxiv]. Yippee! I am certain I have socks in my drawer that are older than that. I've had to contemplate my own mortality a bit more than your average 30-something adult. If your illness is degenerative or incurable, you may be looking at a similar scenario.

I have ways of dealing with this harsh reality that I've gleaned from other survivors. For instance, I tell myself I'm not a statistic. Or, as I mentioned at the beginning of the book, I do remind myself there is no expiration date stamped on the bottom of my foot telling me when my shelf life is up. And these things help.

But the other way I've had to deal with this is simply to come to terms with it. Another patient once asked me if I thought I was going to die soon. As I was doing pretty well, this took me completely by surprise... until he explained that his perception was that I talked about death as if it was imminent. I had to chew on that one for a while. I came to the conclusion that I do indeed address the topic of death pretty head on. Do I intend to be here to see my son graduate from high school, move on to college, someday get married... of course I do! But I've also somehow learned to live for a bright future while acknowledging the more shadowy places that may come, and preparing for them.

It's not so different than buying life insurance, really. You prepare for the worst and hope for the best. It's just that my preparations are a bit more... pressing. I know what songs I want at my funeral, I know what I will leave my son to remember me by. I know what message I want to leave behind. I have faith that I won't need these things in the near future. But, which is worse? Knowing the legacy and message you want to leave behind, and never getting the chance, or facing it and making sure it happens?

And speaking of the worst, you know what's REALLY the worst? The way we talk about those who have passed after an illness. Think about what we always say, *"Oh, she lost her battle with PH. (cancer, Lupus, AIDS, etc)"* Say what???

Think about it. If your neighbor crosses a busy street and meets an unfortunate end, we don't say, "She lost her battle with a speeding bus."

If your grandfather lives to the ripe old age of 97 and passes quietly in his sleep, we don't say, "He lost his battle with aging."

No, of course not. And that sounds ridiculous, doesn't it? So why in heaven's name would we take the strongest, bravest, most dedicated fighters for life, those who have major illness, and decide that once their time has come, they have lost?

I don't believe I have lost anything. Sure, my diagnosis has taken things from me. It might even take more. But, at the end of this, I have not and will not have lost a battle. Not if I fight a good fight, keep my dignity, and keep trying like hell to make a difference. No way. I will have won. My time will simply be up.

So, please, please, if that time comes, do not say you or your friends have lost their battle. Instead, look to the journey as just that, a journey. And celebrate that.

And, unequivocally, can we please collectively agree to stop using the term, "She lost her battle." It is life after all. As far as I know, nobody gets out of life alive.

Healthy people often wonder how I do what I do – how I face a disease that was supposed to take me down with the positive nature and sense of fight I try to emit every day. They tell me they would never have the strength. I tell them you never know what you're capable of until you're forced to step up. And while I'm sure some of what I put forth is just part of who I am, I also believe I got a lot of my spunk from my grandmother.

She was the most amazing woman. Born and bred in New York City, she was an Upper East Side Irish princess who married a rough and tumble Irishman (my grandfather) from the wrong side of the tracks. She could be sweet and loving or raging and swearing like a sailor with equal intensity. While I always deeply loved and admired her, it was her final years that taught me more about living and dying than anything else ever has.

Soon after my grandfather passed while I was still in high school, my parents re-located her from New York to be with us. She lived in our home for a couple of years, transitioned to assisted living, and finally, after a few strokes, to a nursing home. We had her nearby for 13 years, and every time I got to be with her was a blessing.

Her last years, from around ages 90 - 92, were bumpy. She routinely scared the daylights out of us, falling ill, making us think this might be "it", and then bouncing back, punchy as ever. She did this perhaps an easy dozen times, if not more. Sometimes I would wait it out at home, a good four hours from where she lived near my parents. Sometimes I would rush to be by her side. But she always pulled through, and it seemed she could do it forever.

I never told her about my illness. I barred my family from doing so as well. I was so afraid I would break her heart. She loved us grandkids fiercely. *"So what's new?"* she'd always ask. *"You're my best pet"*, she'd often say, patting our arm. I just couldn't imagine responding to that with, *"Grandma, I'm sick... and it isn't good."* I couldn't stand the thought of giving her sadness when I could protect her. After a great deal of time had passed, and I started doing so much better, I just didn't know how to start the conversation. I don't regret hiding it. Truly, I don't. But clearly, she was so strong. I suppose she could have withstood it.

We are much alike. I have her pale blue eyes, her stature (but never her tiny waist), her spunk, and her sharp tongue. And, oh yeah, we even had the same cup size at one point. Go ahead and giggle. I do. But that woman kicked breast cancer to the curb and lived to tell the tale. Just like I intend to kick my own illness. So whatever she had, I'll take it.

In her final month, I had some profound experiences with her. In that nursing home where she had resided for nearly a decade, things began to shift. She had outlived not only nearly 93 years of world events, but also my grandfather's cancer and emphysema and death, followed by her own breast cancer, and back surgery, and multiple strokes. Through it all, she somehow was able to thrive. Her wig was always carefully in place, her eyebrows drawn in pencil, one always slightly higher than the other so it always seemed she was giving you a look. Somebody did her nails – always red. She shared a little cocktail with my dad on Friday afternoons. Ninety-two years old and the woman kept it together against all the odds.

That final weekend visit before the one I took when she died was different. On this weekend I saw what my parents meant by *"Grandma isn't doing so well."* with my own eyes. On this weekend, instead of her greeting us up and in her chair, pulled together as usual, she was in bed, dressed but disoriented. It was clear to me she was dehydrated. I held her frail body upright. My relatively strong arms wrapped around her, holding her up so she could take a sip of much needed water. I changed her shirt... after that sip of water, or a leaky cup, or a faulty straw, or her inability to drink, whatever it was, soaked her shirt to the skin, necessitating a clean one. She didn't have the strength to do it herself.

As I struggled to change her, to lift her meticulously kept clothes over a body bent and broken, as I caught sight of her body, marred by cancer and age, with the prosthetic boob shoved in her bra... the one she took pride in placing, even as she was prone to joke about it and make my dad blush... I was just... struck.

Struck by the fragility of life. Struck by the fact that I, her granddaughter, could hold this old precious woman in my arms and offer her comfort... even as she cursed out the nurse who was "a dope" (a fact on which I concurred), or complained about her roommate who was "off her rack" (also true). While I giggled at her sharp tongue, and admonished her to be nice, I couldn't help but wish that her spark would always be with me as well.

I see so much of myself in her that goes beyond our physical similarities, and beyond our shared middle name. I strive to share her spunk, her will to live, her efforts to maintain her dignity though some nice clothes and a little make-up, no matter how crappy she felt.

My greatest wish was to be there in her final moments. I only wanted to hold her hand, to kiss her forehead goodbye, just as I did every time we said "so long", and to wish her peace in those final moments of her life here on earth. Just a couple of weeks later I would find myself rushing back to be by her side, this time to help usher her home to heaven. It was an incredibly difficult experience. There were moments I had to leave the room to collect myself, and moments I was able to reach and calm her when nothing else would. It was in those moments where I *could* calm her just by my hand on her arm, my head bowed, sending her all the strength and peace I could muster, that I began to first sense the power of energy that can be transferred between two humans. I would go and get certified in Reiki just a few months after that.

When she finally fell into a coma and then breathed her last, her family was around her sending her love. My sister had just returned to the room and as her footsteps hit the floor, Grandma, who it seemed was waiting for us all to be there, simply took a breath and stopped. My dad was holding her hand, my mom at his side, and my sister and I held each other. While there are things about the hours before she died I would do anything to change, the final moments were peaceful and everything we could have hoped for.

I tell you all of this because I wish the same for you and me. The wish is simple. Dignity in the face of illness, strength in the face of whatever comes, surrounded by those you love, and enough spark to put people in their place when they are just plain "dopey". Truly, my grandmother was something to aspire to. If I can emulate her in my final days and moments, it will all be okay.

It seems that to leave this world with a sense of peace, there are some things we need to do in this life to ease the transition into the next. There are the practical things, like living wills and advanced directives, which will ideally serve as a guide on how your care and wishes will be carried out in the final days, and the days that follow. Again, I highly encourage you to speak with your doctor and consult a lawyer on these matters. You don't want room for error, and laws will vary state by state.

But beyond those practicalities, there's still today. In the next chapter I'd like you to take a look at how you live your life now so that when your time does come, whenever that is, however that is, you will know you have lived life right. Specifically, I want you to consider how will you leave your mark on the world? In that case, it doesn't matter where you are in your medical journey. You can start making a difference now, and when your time does come, no matter the cause, you will have left the world a better place. Who knows how far it will take you, and in what ways you can and will leave this world a better place.

Defining Moment

Have you faced your own mortality? It is a difficult thing for many in our culture to do, but so important to spend a little time getting real with what is, in the end, everyone's reality. Try to work on thinking about it in a way that leaves you with at least a little sense of peace.

1) When I think of my passing, what thoughts come to mind?

2) When I think of my passing, are there emotions I struggle with? What are they?

(continued on next page)

3) What little things can I do now to prepare so that when my time does come, I will have left my loved ones with the memories I want them to have? (Write letters, organize pictures, plan your own special touches for a memorial, etc.)

4) Am I okay (emotionally) making these sorts of plans? If not, whom do I need to talk with to start working on a more peaceful feeling around end of life planning? (Pastor, friend, etc.)

CHAPTER 26
The Power of Reaching Out

"My mission in life is not merely to survive, but to thrive; and to do so with some passion, some compassion, some humor, and some style"
~Maya Angelou

What if just by the simple act of reaching out to another patient you could start to feel better? What if your public actions increased awareness, which increased funding for research, which drove your community straight to better treatments and maybe even a cure? What if *you* had that kind of power? What if you DO have this kind of power?

I believe this ripple effect is absolutely possible. In fact, I know it is, because I watch it happen every day.

My friend Katie puts it this way,

"With every breath, with every heart beat, with every step we take, we make an impact on the world around us. We have the power to soothe a broken heart, to shine a light in the darkness of disease. The power of a smile and the gift of laughter can help to lift someone out of the grips of depression. A shoulder to cry on, a hand to hold, a hug to remind us we are loved can be just as powerful as the strongest drugs on the market. No matter what the obstacle - hope, courage, strength, and faith are key factors in coping, in healing the mind, body and soul."[lxxv]

There are really great reasons why I started to get better. The right medications, taking care of myself, and everything we've covered in this book played a part. But I think one of the biggest things that helped me heal was also the one most outside myself – the part where I got out of my own head and out of my own way, and extended a hand to others.

As an extension of that, I quickly found that working hard on advocacy and awareness raising for my disease state gave me a sense of power and control over my outcome. This is when I truly began to become more than my diagnosis. I may not see the cure come, but I will always know I am doing everything possible to help it get here. That alone can help you start to feel a little better!

If you're reading this book, odds are you have a diagnosis that doesn't have a cure. Or maybe there is a cure, but the road is long and hard, and the physical cost high. Either way, I'll bet you're hoping pretty hard for a better answer. I know I am. The thing is, if we have the right to hope for a cure, then each and every one of us has this tremendous responsibility to become a part of the fight that gets us there. When it comes down to it, none of us experience our disease in a vacuum. None of us are on a solitary journey. If we band together in the fight, how much stronger will we be?

I believe each of us has a gift, maybe more than one gift, and if we each tap into our own talents, then a ripple around the world will continue until we each get the cure we all are hoping for. To make a difference in this world, we must become vulnerable, open our hearts and minds, and be ready to bear some of the burden for one another. A combination of passion, compassion, and vulnerability, while incredibly difficult to navigate on some days, can move mountains.

This process of connecting and outreach is not without challenges. Since most of my patient contact is online, and I interact with at least a thousand of them in any given week, that means that time after time I've had to say a virtual and final goodbye to someone who shares my disease. The feeling this evokes is hard to articulate. It is soul shaking. But there came a point in this journey where I both realized it was going to keep happening and deemed it worth it. My community needs me. I need them. The relationship becomes 100% reciprocal.

So, what's *your* gift? Because I know you have one. Whatever it is, be it supporting others, or fundraising, or educating those who can help make a difference in the course of your disease or the funding that gets you there, you need to do it. Better yet, find a group to do it with and see your efforts multiply.

If you haven't spent time considering what your gifts are, now is the time to do so. Let's look at some different ways people can contribute to a cause.

Support Networks: Perhaps you have a gift of connecting with people. We talked a lot about support groups in a different section of this book, but for the sake of this idea of giving back, let's re-visit. When you join a support group, you become a shoulder for others to lean on, and they become that for you. Your story of perseverance is bound to help a newly diagnosed or struggling patient find a glimmer of hope to cling to. Your ability to navigate the health care system and self-advocate (maybe because of skills you learn from this book!), will help another patient find their strong voice in their care. Beyond support groups, you may find that there are organizations that allow you to be an email or phone mentor to others with your condition. Sometimes the greatest gift you can give is a listening ear. Become connected to others and watch what happens when you band together.

Legislative Advocacy Work: Perhaps you have a gift of being able to tell your story well and inspire others to action. We are really blessed to live in a country where our voices still matter. Our elected officials still listen to their constituents because, at the end of the day, our votes still put them in office. Sure, there's a whole lot to say about the current practices funding political races and parties, and how lobbyist have a huge amount of clout in Washington. But do not let these things sway you from raising your voice to those who can take your story to a state or national level.

Your members of Senate and Congress have ways to be reached. If you visit their individual websites, you will find the ways to contact them. If the disease state you have has a national organization, they may have advocacy activities already in process, that you can join. You can arrange a trip to Capitol Hill in Washington, DC and visit in person, or arrange a visit to the representative's state offices when they are in-state. E-mail. Call. Make your voice and story heard.

Having visited my own representatives on Capitol Hill twice, and participated in email and phone campaigns for several years running, I've seen first-hand the success this can bring. Between my work and the hard work of others like me, my state representatives have almost all agreed to co-sponsor a bill specific to Pulmonary Hypertension. This is something I believe they never would have done without the personal connection and meetings we requested. How's that for democracy in action? Pretty cool, I think.

Fundraising: Perhaps you have a gift with event planning or creating what is known as "an ask" for financial support. Some people are amazing at this, and for others, it can feel quite uncomfortable, at least at first.

Can I let you in on a little secret? I once hated fundraising for my cause. I mean I *really* hated it. I would happily throw myself into efforts for someone else but there was a time that I wrote publically on my blog that fundraising for PH was simply not for me. I was excusing myself from the responsibility. My reasons for hating fundraising had little to do with actually doing an event. No, what really bothered me was that I hated asking for help. Before I learned to view the help from others as a gift, I was really uncomfortable saying, *"I need this!"*

I admit I've also struggled to ask friends and family for help because of how I, perhaps mistakenly, wish they'd just magically help on their own. But... life isn't like that. Not because they don't care though. Everyone is pulled in a zillion directions, with a zillion possible things to tug on heartstrings, demand attention, and request or require support. So it's up to me, it's up to you if it's important enough, to lead the charge.
On some days it was still hard for me still to admit that my disease so freaking serious that massive action has to be taken if I, or anyone else with my disease, is to survive it. On some days, it was still hard to admit to myself that I'm here in this world of "the girl who has that diagnosis."

But I had to face that I am indeed here. Until someone hands me a cure, I'm here, and I'm in it deep. So are you. Since many of us have a rare disease, and most of us don't have a cure in hand, it pretty much stands to reason that nobody else is going to step up, unless those of us most directly involved in the community do it ourselves, or at least take the lead (hint-hint). What it comes down to is that the drive to move your cause forward needs to trump your perceived comfort level.

It also helps to understand a little bit about the way medical research is funded. There are many different contributors to research funding: The National Institutes of Health, biotechnology companies, medical device companies, federal and state dollars, and private funds all come into play. Every one of these funding sources come with a set of complex rules and regulations around who can give what to whom and how much and under what circumstances. And the rules are always changing.

The forces at work in the economy and the political climate matter. What politicians deem worth saving, cutting, encouraging, and restricting matter. The challenge is that in the current climate, all of these factors mean that the federal rules on research funding regulations, as well as actual federal dollars being allocated, are getting tighter and tighter. Research labs are seeing their budgets from public funds slashed. You want research towards a cure? You need to help make it happen.

So do what you need to do to get comfortable with fundraising. If you aren't up for leading the charge yourself, connect with those who are and support them from behind the scenes. A strong planning committee makes for the most successful fundraisers.

For me, it was as simple as re-framing my view. I didn't want to ask friends and family for money, and I'm still not crazy about that aspect of fundraising. But I can throw one heck of a party. So, that's what I do. From Zumbathons (*Shake it for PH!*) to a more refined gala, I'm happy to put together a great party and invite people to come have some fun as they join my fight.

Media: Perhaps you have a gift for storytelling – specifically, your story. Reaching out to the media is one of my favorite ways to encourage patients to self-advocate and create awareness. Even on those days where you don't feel much like getting off the couch, or are too busy with just managing life and a diagnosis, you can almost always find time to send an email, make a post, or take 20 minutes on the phone to tell your story to an interested reporter.

Members of the traditional media (newspaper, radio, television) are always looking for personal and local stories to feature. The first thing you want to do is connect with a national organization for your diagnosis, if one exists. They may have pre-packaged information for you to use, scripts, or a staff member with whom you can consult. If you don't have an organization with which to align, or media outreach is not a service they offer, don't worry a bit. There is a great deal you can do on your own.

Do a little research on reporters in your area – who covers the health beat or local interest stories? That's whom you will want to reach out to first if possible. Try to connect your media outreach to an event. It can be as simple as the designated awareness month for your diagnosis, or perhaps a fundraiser you are holding (another plug for the value of a fundraiser – media coverage!). Simply call or email, and let the reporter know what you're working on and why.

Even if you don't have an event in the works, it can be as simple as keeping an eye on local or national interest stories and letting reporters know that *your* story fits in with the given topic of interest. Example topics might be new research or drug approval that your diagnosis is tied to or perhaps something that is already featuring a local hospital or doctor with whom you are affiliated. Nobody is going to know you and your story without you being willing to put it out there, so look for creative ways in which you can do so!

Media coverage can add a significant amount of reach to your awareness and fundraising activities. At the very least, you'll want to think about press releases for any event, and even better, seeing about getting a feature human interest story. I have successfully seen proactive patients get themselves in newspapers, on the radio, and even on television. All it takes is that first ask, and then plenty of polite but persistent follow-up.

Another thing you can do is search for local online publications, some of which will be online components to a print production, and others will be strictly online. Some of these online publications allow you to create an account and blog or create your own press releases, and then you are published. In some cases these are also sent out to subscribers on your behalf. Start with www.onlinenewspapers.com and a more general Internet search for community online newspapers to begin to identify online publications near you.

Along with more traditional media outlets comes the power of social media. You absolutely cannot over-estimate how effective leveraging social media for awareness and outreach can be! Free sites such as Facebook, Twitter, Instagram, and Pinterest (and many more!) all allow you to network and spread your message with ease. Use these platforms to meet likeminded patients and advocates, spread the word on events and awareness activities, and even reach potential donors and advocacy allies.

Blogging: I have come to realize that if we are to reach others with our experience and our message then we then must also be vulnerable in how we put ourselves out to the world. I've maintained a blog on my experiences for a number of years (**www.phandthenewnormal.blogspot.com**). There has been many a time when I have hesitated before hitting "publish", sometimes waiting weeks or even months before I was really ready to put something out there, but in the end I pushed the "publish" button, and it mattered.

It can be really hard to put your deepest feelings before the world and not know where they're landing or how they are perceived. But a few times a year I will get an unexpected email from another patient. They'll tell me my little blog gave them hope as they lay in the hospital newly diagnosed, or showed them that the diagnosis they had been handed was not the end game. When I learn that my words and vulnerability have touched another human being, it makes the moments of deepest discomfort totally worth it. If writing is my gift, then I darn well better use it to the maximum. If you like to write, start a simple blog and see where it goes.

Defining Moment

How will you reach out and make a difference for your diagnosis state, or your community?

1) Are there any ways I am currently involved in outreach and advocacy? If so, how's it going? What are my thoughts on how to refine or expand my efforts?

2) What is one thing I can start doing today to get (more) involved?

3) *Write down three steps you will need to take as you begin to take more action. Do you need to research potential contacts? Find a place to host a fundraiser? Open up a blog? What else?*

Three steps I can take are:

a.

b.

c.

I will take these steps by this date:

(continued on next page)

4) My goal or hope of accomplishment for my new activity level is to:

5) *How will you measure your success? It can be something tangible, like a certain amount of money raised, or it can be less tangible, such as a feeling of satisfaction for having made a difference. Or a combination of both types of measure!*

I will measure success by:

CHAPTER 27
This End is Your Beginning

Contentment: Were there an award for people who come to understand the concept of enough. Good enough. Successful enough. Thin enough. Rich enough. Socially responsible enough. When you have self-respect, you have enough
~Gail Sheehy

We have reached the end of our time together in this book. My prayer is that you found things within its pages that gave you hope, and ideas on how to move forward. I trust you learned a few truths about yourself along the way, and hope that you maybe even experienced a smile or a chuckle once in a while.

If you had some ah-ha moments that have helped you, then the first mission of the book has been accomplished. I'd love to hear about them. If you shook up your life and made some amazing life-changing experiences, then I definitely want to hear about them!

Either way, I am grateful you let me be a part of your journey. Many years ago, just about the time I began to get my feet under me after my diagnosis, I made a vow. If I could help it, no other patient would go through what I went through or take as long to learn what took so much hard time to learn – that life at the point of a diagnosis is not over and that we have so much more control of our outcome than we could dream. It's been true for me, and it can be true for you too.

I also promised myself I would spend as much time as I possibly could documenting what worked and sharing it with others. Likewise, I would watch my community and learn where their pain was and do what I could to create ways to fix it. Finally, I would spend as much time as I could learning from those who are so much wiser than I am, and then try to pass that on to others. This book is, in essence, the collection of all that, at least to date, as there will always be room for more. My challenge to you is to now do the same – take what you've learned, take the time to care for yourself as you need, and pay it forward.

There's no doubt that being dealt a major diagnosis may shake you to your core. There's no doubt that things in your life will have to change. But most importantly, there is no doubt that whatever your medical journey, you are still you, and you are so worth investing in. Believe this and will find your new normal, knowing you can define that new reality for yourself.

It's just going to take a little work. Good luck!

~Colleen

Endnotes

[i] Fox, Michael J., A Funny Thing Happened on the Way to the

[ii] "Bio Individuality," Institute of Integrative Nutrition, accessed August 1, 2014, http://www.integrativenutrition.com/glossary/bioindividuality.

[iii] Pulmonary Hypertension Association, accessed August 11, 2014 http://www.PHAssocation.org.

[iv] *Caring Voice Coalition,* accessed August 11, 2014 http://www.CaringVoice.org.

[v] Kam, Katherine, "What is Palliative Care?," WebMD, reviewed on October 15, 2012, http://www.webmd.com/palliative-care/what-is-palliative-care.

[vi] Oregon State University. "Gut microbes closely linked to proper immune function, other health issues." ScienceDaily, accessed August 15, 2014, www.sciencedaily.com/releases/2013/09/130916122214.htm.

[vii] Li, James T., M.D., Ph.D., "What's the difference between a food intolerance and a food allergy?" Mayo Clinic, June 3, 2011, http://www.mayoclinic.org/diseases-conditions/food-allergy/expert-answers/food-allergy/FAQ-20058538.

[viii] de Punder, Karin; Pruimboom, Leo. "The Dietary Intake of Wheat and other Cereal Grains and Their Role in Inflammation," NUTRIENTS 2013 5(3), 771-787; doi:10.3390/nu5030771.

[ix] Foster, Jane A., "Gut Feelings: Bacteria and the Brain," The Dana Foundation, last modified July 1, 2013, http://dana.org/Cerebrum/Default.aspx?id=39496.

[x] The Gaps Diet, accessed August 11, 2014, http://www.gapsdiet.com/.

xi The Body Ecology Diet, accessed August 11, 2014, http://bodyecology.com/.

xii Bein, Barbara, "Medical Schools Struggle to Provide Ample Training in Nutrition, Obesity Prevention," The American Academy of Family Physicians, March 17, 2010, http://www.aafp.org/news/obesity/20100517med-schools.html.

xiii Bellatti, Andy, "The High Cost of Sitting Down with Industry," The Huffington Post, last modified August 8, 2013, http://www.huffingtonpost.com/andy-bellatti/healthy-living-news_b_5673277.html.

xiv Hoffman, Beth, "What Should You Eat? Report Says 'Big Food' Influencing Dieticians," Forbes.com, last modified January 1, 2013, http://www.forbes.com/sites/bethhoffman/2013/01/24/what-should-you-eat-report-says-big-food-influencing-dieticians/.

xv "Overweight and Obesity," Center for Disease Control and Prevention, Last updated September 9, 2014, http://www.cdc.gov/obesity/data/adult.html.

xvi Dr. Mark Hyman, accessed August 12, 2014, http://drhyman.com/.

xvii Dr. Andrew Weil, accessed August 12, 2014, http://www.drweil.com/.

xviii Socha, Katarzyna, et al, "Dietary Habits and Selenium, Glutathione Peroxidase and Total Antioxidant Status in the Serum of Patients with Relapse-Remitting Multiple Sclerosis," NUTRITION JOURNAL 2014, 13:62 doi:10.1186/1475-2891-13-62.

xix Strickland, Faith M., et al, "Diet Influences Expression of Autoimmune Associated Genes and Disease Severity By Epigenetic Mechanisms in a Transgenic Lupus Model." Arthritis Rheum. July 2013; 65(7); 1872-1881. Doi: 10.1002/art.37967.

[xx] "Bio Individuality," Institute of Integrative Nutrition, accessed August 1, 2014, http://www.integrativenutrition.com/glossary/bioindividuality.

[xxi] Pollan, Michael, "Unhappy Meals," The Times Magazine, Last updated January 28, 2007. http://www.nytimes.com/2007/01/28/magazine/28nutritionism.t.html

[xxii] "The New (Ab)Normal: Portion Sizes Today vs. the 1950s," Huffington Post, last updated May 23, 2012, http://www.huffingtonpost.com/2012/05/23/portion-sizes-infographic_n_1539804.html.

[xxiii] "The Protein Myth", Physicians Committee for Responsible Medicine, accessed August 6, 2014, http://www.pcrm.org/health/diets/vegdiets/how-can-i-get-enough-protein-the-protein-myth

[xxiv] Hunt, Chris, "The Arsenic in Your Chicken," The Huffington Post, last updated July 13, 2013, http://www.huffingtonpost.com/chris-hunt/arsenic-in-chicken_b_3267334.html.

[xxv] Geer, Abigail, "10 Things Everyone Should Know About Factory Farmed Animals," *Care2.com, l*ast updated March 27, 2014, http://www.care2.com/causes/10-things-everyone-should-know-about-factory-farmed-animals.html.

[xxvi] Mercola, Joseph, "Coconut oil vs. Vegetable Oil: Which Should You be Cooking With? And Which Should You Avoid?," Mercola.com, last updated October 15, 2003, http://articles.mercola.com/sites/articles/archive/2003/10/15/cooking-oil.aspx.

[xxvii] Campbell-McBride, Natasha. "Gut and Psychology Syndrome: Natural Treatment for Autism, Dyspraxia, A.D.D., Dyslexia, A.D.H.D., Depression, Schizophrenia." (Medinform Publishing, 2010), 53-54.

xxviii "Protein Content of Green Vegetables Compared to Meat?," Dr. Fuhrman.com, accessed August 15, 2014, http://www.drfuhrman.com/faq/question.aspx?sid=16&qindex=9

xxix "Dietary Fat," *Centers for Disease Control and Prevention,* last updated September 27, 2012, http://www.cdc.gov/nutrition/everyone/basics/fat/.

xxx "FDA Takes Step to Further Reduce Trans Fats in Processed Foods," Us Food and Drug Administration, last updated November 7, 2014, http://www.fda.gov/NewsEvents/Newsroom/PressAnnouncements/ucm373939.htm.

xxxi DiSalvo, David, "What Eating too Much Sugar Does to Your Brain," *Psychology Today,* last updated April 27, 2012, http://www.psychologytoday.com/blog/neuronarrative/201204/what-eating-too-much-sugar-does-your-brain

xxxii "Frequently Asked Questions About Sugar," American Heart Association, last updated May 19, 2012, http://www.heart.org/HEARTORG/GettingHealthy/NutritionCenter/HealthyEating/Frequently-Asked-Questions-About-Sugar_UCM_306725_Article.jsp

xxxiii Walton, Alice G., "How Much Sugar Are Americans Eating?," Forbes.com, last updated August 30, 2012, http://www.forbes.com/sites/alicegwalton/2012/08/30/how-much-sugar-are-americans-eating-infographic/.

xxxiv "Concern Over Canned Foods," *ConsumerReports.org,* last updated December 2009, http://www.consumerreports.org/cro/magazine-archive/december-2009/food/bpa/overview/bisphenol-a-ov.htm.

[xxxv] Albaugh, Jeffery A., "Sprituality and Life-Threatening Illness: A Phenomenologic Study," Oncology Nursing Forum. 30(4):593-598, 2003, http://www.ncbi.nlm.nih.gov/pubmed/12861320

[xxxvi] "Spirituality and Chronic Illness," *Montana State University,* Last updated June 14, 2011, http://www.montana.edu/cweinert/spichronic.html.

[xxxvii] Johnson, Bonnie, E-mail message to the author, August 28, 2014.

[xxxviii] Epstein, Bert H., "15 Ways to Get a Good Night's Sleep," *Oregon State University,* accessed September 1, 2014, http://oregonstate.edu/counsel/15-ways-get-good-nights-sleep

[xxxix] Sutter, John D., "Trouble Sleeping? Maybe it's your iPad." *CNN.com.* Last updated May 13, 2010. http://www.cnn.com/2010/TECH/05/13/sleep.gadgets.ipad/index.html.

[xl] "A Great Night's Sleep Can Depend on the Visual Conditions in Your Bedroom Environment," *SleepFoundation.org*, accessed August 16, 2014, http://sleepfoundation.org/bedroom/see.php.

[xli] Cuda, Gretchen, "Just Breathe: Body Has a Built-in Stress Reliever," *National Public Radio,* last updated December 6, 2010, http://www.npr.org/2010/12/06/131734718/just-breathe-body-has-a-built-in-stress-reliever.

[xlii] Aroma Tools, Modern Essentials: A Contemporary Guide to Therapeutic Use of Essential Oils (The NEW 5th Edition), Aroma Tools, 2013. 74 – 75, 100 – 101, 104 - 105

[xliii] "Aromatherapy," University of Maryland Medical Center, last updated August 9, 2011, http://umm.edu/health/medical/altmed/treatment/aromatherapy.

xliv Marten, Galen, telephone interview with the author, September 1, 2014.

xlv Aldis, Barbara, "A New Remedy for Patients Suffering From Lung Conditions: Take up Singing!," MailOnline, last updated May 14, 2013, http://www.dailymail.co.uk/health/article-2324098/A-new-remedy-patients-suffering-lung-conditions-Take-singing.html

xlvi Horn,Stacy, "Singing Changes Your Brain," Time, last updated August 16, 2013, http://ideas.time.com/2013/08/16/singing-changes-your-brain/

xlvii Ottaway, Lynn, Facebook interview with the author, September 2, 2014.

xlviii Pacelli, Jhenna, Facebook interview with the author, September 3, 2014.

xlix "100 Art Therapy Exercises – The Updated and Improved List, " Expressive Art Inspirations, accessed September 1, 2014, http://intuitivecreativity.typepad.com/expressiveartinspirations/100-art-therapy-exercises.html.

l Vogel, Carol, "A Pollock is Sold, Possibly for a Record Price," *The New York Times.* Last updated November 2, 2014, http://www.nytimes.com/2006/11/02/arts/design/02drip.html?_r=2&
li *Funky Folk Art by KVO*, accessed September 17, 2014, http://www.funkyfolkartbykvo.com/
lii Van Osdale-Levitt, Kathy, Interview with Colleen Brunetti, Personal Interview, Facebook, September 2, 2014.

liii Grate, Rachel, "Science Shows Something Surprising About People Who Write," Mic.com, last updated September 15, 2014, http://mic.com/articles/98348/science-shows-writers-have-a-serious-advantage-over-the-rest-of-us.

liv Lynn, Haley-Ann, Facebook interview with the author, September 20, 2014.

lv "What is Trauma?," The Center for Nonviolence and Social Justice, accessed September 4, 2014, http://www.nonviolenceandsocialjustice.org/FAQs/What-is-Trauma/41/.

lvi Tuckman, E-mail and phone call with the author, September 3, 2014.

lvii "What Causes Depression?," Harvard Health Publications, accessed September 17, 2014, http://www.health.harvard.edu/newsweek/what-causes-depression.htm.

lviii Studer, Sean, et al, "The Impact of Pulmonary Arterial Hypertension (PAH) on the Lives of Patients and Caregivers: Results from a U.S. Study," PHA Online University, accessed September 1, 2014, http://www.phaonlineuniv.org/DiagnosisTreatment/content.cfm?ItemNumber=3416

lix Feinstein, A., et al, "The Link Between Multiple Sclerosis and Depression." Nature Reviews Neurology. 2014 Sep;10(9):507-17. doi: 10.1038/nrneurol.2014.139.

lx Rathbun, AM, et al, "A Description of Patient and Rheumatologist-Reported Depression Symptoms in an American Rheumatoid Arthritis Registry Population," *Clinical and Experimental Rheumatology Online,* 2014 Jul-Aug;32(4):523-32.

lxi "What is Depression?," National Institute of Mental Health, accessed September 1, 2014, http://www.nimh.nih.gov/health/publications/depression/index.shtml#pub1

lxii "What is Depression?," National Institute of Mental Health, accessed September 1, 2014, http://www.nimh.nih.gov/health/publications/depression/index.shtml#pub10

[lxiii] Ramirez, Diane. Phone conversation with the author. Date unknown.

[lxiv] Aroma Tools, Modern Essentials: A Contemporary Guide to Therapeutic Use of
Essential Oils (The NEW 5th Edition), Aroma Tools, 2013, 183.

[lxv] Aroma Tools, Modern Essentials: A Contemporary Guide to Therapeutic Use of
Essential Oils (The NEW 5th Edition), Aroma Tools, 2013, 208.

[lxvi] "Harvard Open Courses: Open Learning Initiative," *Harvard Extension School,* Accessed September 17, 2014, http://www.extension.harvard.edu/open-learning-initiative.

[lxvii] Lazzaro, Ronald, Personal Interview with the author, September 24, 2014.

[lxviii] Roberts, Dorothy, Facebook interview with the author, June 27, 2014.

[lxix] Kohler, Jessie, E-mail interview with the author, September 16, 2014.

[lxx] Brunetti, Colleen, Busam, Samantha, "Helping Your Healthy Child Cope With Your Illness," Pulmonary Hypertension Association, last Updated April, 2012, http://www.phassociation.org/HelpingHealthyKidsCope.

[lxxi] Farrow, Patty. Facebook interview with the author. June 26, 2014.

[lxxii] Taylor, Doug. E-mail interview with the author. July 29, 2014.

[lxxiii] "Young Adults with PH", accessed September 15, 2014, http://www.phassociation.org/Patients/YoungAdults.

[lxxiv] McGoon, Michael, Miller, D.P., "REVEAL: A Contemporary US Pulmonary Arterial

Hypertension Registry." European Respiratory Update. 2012; 21: 123, 8–18 DOI: 10.1183/09059180.00008211

[76] Tobias, Katie, interview with the author, August 1, 2014.

Bibliography

"100 Art Therapy Exercises – The Updated and
Improved List." *Expressive Art
Inspirations.* Accessed September 1, 2014.
http://intuitivecreativity.typepad.com/expressiveartinspirations/100-
art-therapy-exercises.html.

"A Great Night's Sleep Can Depend on the Visual Conditions in
Your Bedroom
Environment." *SleepFoundation.org.* Accessed August 16, 2014.
http://sleepfoundation.org/bedroom/see.php.

"Aromatherapy." *University of Maryland Medical Center.*
Last updated August 9, 2011.
http://umm.edu/health/medical/altmed/treatment/aromatherapy.

Albaugh, Jeffery A. "Sprituality and Life-Threatening
Illness: A Phenomenologic Study."
Oncology Nursing Forum. 30(4):593-598, 2003.
http://www.ncbi.nlm.nih.gov/pubmed/12861320

Aldis, Barbara. "A New Remedy for Patients Suffering
From Lung Conditions: Take up
Singing!." *MailOnline.* Last updated May 14, 2013.
http://www.dailymail.co.uk/health/article-2324098/A-new-remedy-
patients-
suffering-lung-conditions-Take-singing.html

Aroma Tools. Modern Essentials: A Contemporary Guide
to Therapeutic Use of
Essential Oils (The NEW 5th Edition). Aroma Tools, 2013. 74 – 75,
100 – 101, 104 – 105, 183, 208

Bein, Barbara. "Medical Schools Struggle to Provide
Ample Training in Nutrition,
Obesity Prevention." *The American Academy of Family Physicians.*
Last modified March 17, 2010.
http://www.aafp.org/news/obesity/20100517med-schools.html.

Bellatti, Andy. "The High Cost of Sitting Down with
Industry." *The Huffington Post.*
Last modified August 8, 2013. http://www.huffingtonpost.com/andy-
bellatti/healthy-living-news_b_5673277.html.

"Bio Individuality." *Institute of Integrative Nutrition.*
accessed August 1, 2014,
http://www.integrativenutrition.com/glossary/bioindividuality.

Brunetti, Colleen, Busam, Samantha. "Helping Your
Healthy Child Cope With Your
Illness." *Pulmonary Hypertension Association.* Last Updated April,
2012. http://www.phassociation.org/HelpingHealthyKidsCope.

Caring Voice Coalition, Accessed August 11, 2014.
http://www.CaringVoice.org.

Campbell-McBride, Natasha. "Gut and Psychology
Syndrome: Natural Treatment for
Autism, Dyspraxia, A.D.D., Dyslexia, A.D.H.D., Depression,
Schizophrenia." Medinform Publishing, 2010, 56-59.

"Concern Over Canned Foods." *ConsumerReports.org.*
Last updated December 2009.
http://www.consumerreports.org/cro/magazine-archive/december-
2009/food/bpa/overview/bisphenol-a-ov.htm

Cuda, Gretchen. "Just Breathe: Body Has a Built-in
Stress Reliever." *National Public
Radio.* Last updated December 6, 2010.
http://www.npr.org/2010/12/06/131734718/just-breathe-body-has-a-
built-in-stress-reliever.

"Dietary Fat." *Centers for Disease Control and Prevention.* Last updated September 27, 2012. http://www.cdc.gov/nutrition/everyone/basicsat/.

DiSalvo, David. "What Eating too Much Sugar Does to Your Brain." *Psychology Today.* Last updated April 27, 2012. http://www.psychologytoday.com/blog/neuronarrative/201204/what-eating-too-much-sugar-does-your-brain

de Punder, Karin; Pruimboom, Leo. "The Dietary Intake of Wheat and other Cereal Grains and Their Role in Inflammation." *NUTRIENTS 2013* 5(3), 771-787; doi:10.3390/nu5030771.

Dr. Andrew Weil, accessed August 12, 2014, http://www.drweil.com/.

Dr. Mark Hyman. Accessed August 12, 2014. http://drhyman.com/.

Faith M. Strickland, Anura Hewagama, Ailing Wu, Amr. H. Sawalha, Colin Delaney, Mark F. Hoelzel, Raymond Yung, Kent Johnson, Barbara Mickelson, and Bruce C. Richardson. "Diet Influences Expression of Autoimmune Associated Genes and Disease Severity by Epigenetic Mechanisms in Transgenic Lupus Model." Arthritis Rheum. July 2013; 65(7); 1872-1881. Doi: 10.1002/art.37967.

Farrow, Patty. Facebook interview with the author. June 26, 2014.

"FDA Takes Step to Further Reduce Trans Fats in Processed Foods." *Us Food and Drug Administration.* Last updated November 7, 2014. http://www.fda.gov/NewsEvents/Newsroom/PressAnnouncements/ucm373939.htm

Foster, Jane A. "Gut Feelings: Bacteria and the Brain."
The Dana Foundation, last modified July 1, 2013.
http://dana.org/Cerebrum/Default.aspx?id=39496.

Fox, Michael J., A Funny Thing Happened on the Way to
the Future (Kindle Edition,
2010).

"Frequently Asked Questions About Sugar." *American
Heart Association.* Last updated May 19, 2012.
http://www.heart.org/HEARTORG/GettingHealthy/NutritionCenter/
HealthyEating/Frequently-Asked-Questions-About-
Sugar_UCM_306725_Article.jsp.

Geer, Abigail. "10 Things Everyone Should Know
About Factory Farmed Animals."

Care2.com. Last updated March 27, 2014.
http://www.care2.com/causes/10-things-everyone-should-know-
about-factory-farmed-animals.html.

Grate, Rachel. "Science Shows Something Surprising
About People Who Write."
Mic.com. Last updated September 15, 2014.
http://mic.com/articles/98348/science-shows-writers-have-a-serious-
advantage-over-the-rest-of-us

"Harvard Open Courses: Open Learning Initiative."
Harvard Extension School. Accessed
September 17, 2014. http://www.extension.harvard.edu/open-
learning-initiative.

Hoffman, Beth. "What Should You Eat? Report Says
'Big Food' Influencing Dieticians."
Forbes.com. Last modified January 1, 2013.
http://www.forbes.com/sites/bethhoffman/2013/01/24/what-should-
you-eat-report-says-big-food-influencing-dieticians/.

Horn, Stacy. "Singing Changes Your Brain." Time. Last updated August 16, 2013. http://ideas.time.com/2013/08/16/singing-changes-your-brain/

Hunt, Chris. "The Arsenic in Your Chicken." *The Huffington Post.* Last updated July 13, 2013. http://www.huffingtonpost.com/chris-hunt/arsenic-in-chicken_b_3267334.html.

Kohler, Jessie. E-mail interview with the author. September 16, 2014.

Epstein, Bert H., "15 Ways to Get a Good Night's Sleep." *Oregon State University.* Accessed September 1, 2014. http://oregonstate.edu/counsel/15-ways-get-good-nights-sleep

Feinstein, A., Magalhaes, S., Richard, JF., Audet B., Moore, C., "The Link Between Multiple Sclerosis and Depression." *Nature Reviews Neurology.* 2014 Sep;10(9):507-17. doi: 10.1038/nrneurol.2014.139.

Funky Folk Art by KVO. Accessed September 17, 2014. http://www.funkyfolkartbykvo.com/

Johnson, Bonnie. E-mail message to the author. August 28, 2014.

Kam, Katherine. "What is Palliative Care?." *WebMD.* Reviewed on October 15, 2012. http://www.webmd.com/palliative-care/what-is-palliative-care.

Katarzyna Socha, Jan Kochanowicz, Elżbieta
Karpińska, Jolanta Soroczyńska, Marta
Jakoniuk, Zenon Mariak· and Maria H Borawska. "Dietary Habits
and Selenium, Glutathione Peroxidase and Total Antioxidant Status
in the Serum of Patients with Relapse-Remitting Multiple Sclerosis."
NUTRITION JOURNAL 2014, 13:62 doi:10.1186/1475-2891-13-62.

Lazzaro, Ronald. Personal Interview with the author.
September 24, 2014.

Li, James T., M.D., Ph.D. "What's the difference
between a food intolerance and a food
allergy?." *Mayo Clinic.* June 3, 2011.
http://www.mayoclinic.org/diseases-conditions/food-allergy/expert-
answers/food-allergy/FAQ-20058538.

Lynn, Haley-Ann. Facebook interview with the author.
September 20, 2014.

Marten, Galen. Telephone interview with the author.
September 1, 2014.

Mercola, Joseph. "Coconut oil vs. Vegetable Oil: Which
Should You be Cooking With? And Which Should You Avoid?."
Mercola.com. Last updated October 15, 2003.
http://articles.mercola.com/sites/articles/archive/2003/10/15/cooking
-oil.aspx.

Oregon State University. "Gut microbes closely linked
to proper immune function, other
health issues." *ScienceDaily,.* Accessed August 15,
2014.www.sciencedaily.com/releases/2013/09/130916122214.htm.

Ottaway, Lynn. Facebook interview with the author.
September 2, 2014.

"Overweight and Obesity." *Center for Disease Control and Prevention*. Last updated September 9, 2014. http://www.cdc.gov/obesity/data/adult.html.

McGoon, Michael, Miller, D.P., "REVEAL: A Contemporary US Pulmonary Arterial Hypertension Registry." *European Respiratory Update*. 2012; 21: 123, 8–18 DOI: 10.1183/09059180.00008211

Pacelli, Jhenna. Facebook interview with the author. September 3, 2014.

Pollan, Michael. "Unhappy Meals.", *The Times Magazine*. Last updated January 28, 2007. http://www.nytimes.com/2007/01/28/magazine/28nutritionism.t.html

"Protein Content of Green Vegetables Compared to Meat?." *Dr. Fuhrman.com*. Accessed August 15, 2014. http://www.drfuhrman.com/faq/question.aspx?sid=16&qindex=9.

Pulmonary Hypertension Association Accessed August 11, 2014. http://www.PHAssociation.org.

Ramirez, Diane. Phone conversation with the author. Date unknown.

Rathbun, AM, Harrold LR, Reed GW. "A Description of Patient and Rheumatologist-Reported Depression Symptoms in an American Rheumatoid Arthritis Registry Population." *Clinical and Experimental Rheumatology Online*. 2014 Jul-Aug;32(4):523-32.

Roberts, Dorothy. Facebook interview with the author. June 27, 2014.

"Spirituality and Chronic Illness." *Montana State University.* Last updated June 14, 2011.
http://www.montana.edu/cweinert/spichronic.html.
Sutter, John D., "Trouble Sleeping? Maybe it's your iPad." *CNN.com.* Last updated May 13, 2010.
http://www.cnn.com/2010/TECH/05/13/sleep.gadgets.ipad/index.html.

The Body Ecology Diet. Accessed August 11, 2014.
http://bodyecology.com/.

Studer, Sean, Deb McCollister, Hubert Chen, Sandra Lombardi, Mary Mullen, Aryeh Fisher, Rino Aldreghetti, Myung Park. "The Impact of Pulmonary Arterial Hypertension (PAH) on the Lives of Patients and Caregivers: Results from a U.S. Study." *PHA Online University.* Accessed September 1, 2014.
http://www.phaonlineuniv.org/DiagnosisTreatment/content.cfm?ItemNumber=3416

Taylor, Doug. E-mail interview with the author. July 29, 2014.

The Gaps Diet. Accessed August 11, 2014.
http://www.gapsdiet.com/.

"The New (Ab)Normal: Portion Sizes Today vs. the 1950s." *Huffington Post.* Last updated May 23, 2012.
http://www.huffingtonpost.com/2012/05/23/portion-sizes-infographic_n_1539804.html.

"The Protein Myth." *Physicians Committee for Responsible Medicine.* Accessed August 6, 2014.
http://www.pcrm.org/health/diets/vegdiets/how-can-i-get-enough-protein-the-protein-myth.

Tobias, Katie. Facebook interview with the author. August 1, 2014.

Tuckman, Rachel. E-mail and phone call interview with the author. September 3, 2014.

"Young Adults with PH". Accessed September 15. *Pulmonary Hypertension Association.* 2014.http://www.phassociation.org/Patients/YoungAdults.

Vogel, Carol. "A Pollock is Sold, Possibly for a Record Price." *The New York Times.* Last updated November 2, 2014. http://www.nytimes.com/2006/11/02/arts/design/02drip.html?_r=2&

Van Osdale-Levitt, Kathy. Facebook interview with author. September 2, 2014.

Walton, Alice G. "How Much Sugar Are Americans Eating?." *Forbes.com.* Last updated August 30, 2012. http://www.forbes.com/sites/alicegwalton/2012/08/30/how-much-sugar-are-americans-eating-infographic/.

"What Causes Depression?." *Harvard Health Publications.* Accessed September 17, 2014.http://www.health.harvard.edu/newsweek/what-causes-depression.htm.

"What is Depression?." *National Institute of Mental Health.* Accessed September 1, 2014.http://www.nimh.nih.gov/health/publications/depression/index.shtml#pub1.

"What is Trauma?." *The Center for Nonviolence and Social Justice.* Accessed September 4, 2014. http://www.nonviolenceandsocialjustice.org/FAQs/What-is-Trauma/41/.

Made in the USA
San Bernardino, CA
28 October 2014